ATLAS OF TIME LAPSE EMBRYOLOGY

EDITED BY

Alison Campbell, BSc(Hons), MMedSci, Dip RC Path
Head of Embryology, CARE Fertility Group, Nottingham, UK

Simon Fishel, PhD
Managing Director, CARE Fertility Group, Nottingham, UK

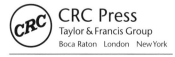

CRC Press
Taylor & Francis Group
Boca Raton London New York

CRC Press is an imprint of the
Taylor & Francis Group, an **informa** business

CRC Press
Taylor & Francis Group
6000 Broken Sound Parkway NW, Suite 300
Boca Raton, FL 33487-2742

© 2015 by Taylor & Francis Group, LLC
CRC Press is an imprint of Taylor & Francis Group, an Informa business

No claim to original U.S. Government works

Printed on acid-free paper
Version Date: 20140818

International Standard Book Number-13: 978-1-4822-1446-8 (Pack - Book and Ebook)

Library of Congress Cataloging-in-Publication Data

Atlas of time lapse embryology / editors, Simon Fishel, Alison Campbell.
  p. ; cm.
  Includes bibliographical references and index.
  ISBN 978-1-4822-1446-8 (alk. paper)
  I. Fishel, S. (Simon) II. Campbell, Alison, 1970-
  [DNLM: 1. Fertilization in Vitro--Atlases. 2. Ectogenesis--Atlases. 3. Embryonic Development--Atlases. 4. Time-Lapse Imaging--Atlases. WQ 17]

RG135
618.1'780599--dc23   2014028482

Visit the Taylor & Francis Web site at
http://www.taylorandfrancis.com

and the CRC Press Web site at
http://www.crcpress.com

ATLAS OF
TIME LAPSE
EMBRYOLOGY

Contents

Contributors..vii

Acknowledgements...ix

Introduction...xi

Videos..xiii

1   EQUIPMENT REQUIRED FOR TIME LAPSE OBSERVATIONS IN IN VITRO FERTILIZATION..............................1
    Louise Best

2   CLINICAL ASPECTS OF TIME LAPSE IMAGING 7
    Alison Campbell

3   TIME LAPSE, THE CELL CYCLE, DISTRIBUTION OF MORPHOKINETIC TIMINGS, AND KNOWN
    IMPLANTATION DATA..13
    Alison Campbell

4   GENDER AND MORPHOKINETICS CORRELATION 19
    Samantha Duffy

5   POLAR-BODY EXTRUSION..21
    Colleen Lynch and Mercedes Regueira

6   FERTILIZATION: PRONUCLEAR FORMATION AND FADING 25
    Louise Kellam and Laina Murphy

7   CLINICAL RESULTS: DYNAMIC ASPECTS – FRAGMENTATION 33
    Sue Montgomery

8   NUMBER OF PRONUCLEI AND PLOIDY IN IVF/ICSI–DERIVED EMBRYOS 39
    Abigail A. Burchill

9   DYNAMIC ASPECTS: COMPACTION 43
    Sue Montgomery

10 BLASTULATION 49
    Sue Montgomery

11 HATCHING OF THE HUMAN BLASTOCYST 59
    Louise Kellam

12 IRREGULAR CLEAVAGES 65
    Kathryn Berrisford and Ellen Cater

13 REVERSE CLEAVAGE/BLASTOMERE FUSION..69
    Davina Hulme

14 SMOOTH ENDOPLASMIC RETICULUM CLUSTERS 71
    Cath Drezet

15 MULTINUCLEATION 75
    Claire Shearer

16 VACUOLATION 79
    Rachel Smith

17   GRANULAR CYTOPLASM..89
      Sarah Foley

18   ZONA DEFECTS 95
      Gerri Emerson

19   THE PATIENT PERSPECTIVE.. 115
      Samantha Duffy

Index... 119

Contributors

Kathryn Berrisford, BSc (Hons)
CARE Fertility
Nottingham, United Kingdom

Louise Best, BSc (Hons)
CARE Fertility
Manchester, United Kingdom

Abigail A. Burchill, BSc (Hons), MMedSci
CARE Fertility
Sheffield, United Kingdom

Alison Campbell, BSc (Hons), MMedSci, Dip RC Path
CARE Fertility
Nottingham, United Kingdom

Ellen Cater BSc (Hons)
CARE Fertility
Nottingham, United Kingdom

Cath Drezet, BSc
CARE Fertility
Sheffield, United Kingdom

Samantha Duffy, BSc (Hons)
CARE Fertility
Manchester, United Kingdom

Gerri Emerson, MSc (Hons), Dip RC Path
Beacon CARE Fertility
Dublin, Ireland

Sarah Foley, BSc (Hons), MSc
CARE Fertility
Sheffield, United Kingdom

Davina Hulme, BSc (Hons), MMedSci
CARE Fertility
Nottingham, United Kingdom

Louise Kellam, BSc (Hons), Dip RC Path
CARE Fertility
Nottingham, United Kingdom

Colleen Lynch, BSc (Hons), MSc
CARE Fertility
Nottingham, United Kingdom

Sue Montgomery, PhD, Dip RC Path
CARE Fertility
Manchester, United Kingdom

Laina Murphy, BSc (Hons)
CARE Fertility
Nottingham, United Kingdom

Mercedes Regueira, BSc, MSc
CARE Fertility
Nottingham, United Kingdom

Claire Shearer, BSc (Hons)
CARE Fertility
Sheffield, United Kingdom

Rachel Smith, BSc (Hons), Dip RC Path
CARE Fertility
Sheffield, United Kingdom

Acknowledgements

We wish to convey our gratitude to CRC Press for the invitation to be involved in this exciting and novel project. We especially thank Keith Tansley for all his dedicated support with image preparation, and all of the authors for their commitment and contributions to this project. We are also very grateful to all members of the CARE Fertility team, who in many different ways have been supportive and instrumental in enabling this unique text to be published. Finally, we express our sincere appreciation to Louise Kellam, who has not only contributed to this Atlas, as an author, but has played a key role in coordinating the submissions between the many other contributors, the editors, and the publisher. Louise Kellam has also taken the lead in developing the image library as a crucial resource for this Atlas and for CARE Fertility embryologists present and future.

Introduction

Since the 1970s and the birth of the world's first IVF baby, Louise Brown, there have been several incremental technological advances affecting clinical embryology, such as advancements in culture media and ambient incubation conditions, and the occasional revolution, such as ICSI and embryo biopsy. Arguably, such advances offer improved treatment for specific patient groups who would otherwise have remained childless. During the last few years, a new technology has become available which already is delivering significant information on the dynamics of cleaving human preimplantation embryos cultured in vitro; and, importantly, evidence is gathering for quantifiable uplifts in the incidence of pregnancy. This technology includes the introduction of safe, sealed incubation systems, where the embryos can remain untouched for several days whilst being monitored by high-frequency time lapse imaging. The ability to acquire sequential, photographic, time lapse images of patients' embryos is fast becoming a powerful, non-invasive embryo monitoring and selection tool. Although 'time lapse cinematography' was used to study fertilization and early human embryo kinetics more than 15 years ago, this technology is now possible using commercially available sophisticated systems for the routine clinical IVF setting which are described in Chapter 1.[1]

An increasing number of publications using time lapse imaging report prognostic markers for embryo viability and implantation potential based on morphokinetic variables. As this technology becomes more widespread a variety of selection models, or algorithms, are being developed.[2–5] Finding a universal model that maximizes the chance for selecting the most viable embryo, and establishing whether such models developed in one setting are effectively transferable to another, remain immediate goals for clinical research. Outcome measures for morphokinetic-based embryo selection models have ranged from blastulation to live birth and have also correlated with embryo ploidy successful implantation and live birth. The prospective use of such models, and the ability to deselect embryos due to cleavage anomalies, has the potential to enhance clinical outcome.

This Atlas, the first of its kind, introduces the general concepts of time lapse imaging and the devices and practice involved, and considers the changing patterns of developmental events associated within the in vitro culture environment – enhancing our knowledge gained from the past, in which embryos were observed using static images, to a new era of dynamic imaging. Within each section of this Atlas, both published and new quantifiable time lapse observations are provided with sequential images supported by descriptive text for clinical examples from a cohort of over nine thousand preimplantation human embryos. The Atlas concludes by considering the IVF patient and presents the patient perspective, looking at questions such as what time lapse imaging meant to them and how they felt about the time lapse video images of their developing embryos, which were made available for them to see.

We hope this Atlas will be instructive to all IVF practitioners hoping to introduce this exciting technology into their IVF practice, and we anticipate the large, collective experience of the CARE Fertility embryology team incorporated in this corpus will aid those embryologists wishing to learn more about the preimplantation human embryo in its dynamic state.

Alison Campbell and Simon Fishel

REFERENCES

1. Payne D, Flaherty SP, Barry MF, Matthews CD. Preliminary observations on polar body extrusion and pronuclear formation in human oocytes using time-lapse video cinematography. *Hum Reprod.* 1997;12:532–41.
2. Wong CC, Loewke KE, Bossert NL, et al. Non-invasive imaging of human embryos before embryonic genome activation predicts development to the blastocyst stage. *Nat Biotechnol.* 2010;28(10):111–1121.
3. Meseguer M, Herrero J, Tejera A, et al. The use of morphokinetics as a predictor of embryo implantation. *Hum Reprod.* 2011:26(10);2658–2671.
4. Campbell A, Fishel S, Bowman N, et al. Modelling a risk classification of aneuploidy in human embryos using non-invasive morphokinetics. *Reprod BioMed Online.* 2013;26:477–485.
5. Basile N, Nogales M, Bronet F, et al. Increasing the probability of selecting chromosomally normal embryos by time-lapse morphokinetics analysis. *Fertil Steril.* 2014 Mar;101(3):699–704.

Videos

Videos cited in *Atlas of Time Lapse Embryology* are accompanied by the following video camera icon: 📹. Corresponding URLs can be found both here and in the chapter text.

Video number	Description	URL
3.1	Oocyte post ICSI as it undergoes fertilization and cell division to a hatching blastocyst. The video pauses at the described morphokinetic time points; t0 is normally considered as the time at insemination (ICSI).	http://goo.gl/U6TN1n
5.1	Development of a 3PN with 1PB.	http://goo.gl/ixaDhA
5.2	Second polar-body extrusion, cytoplasmic movements, and pronuclear formation and fading.	http://goo.gl/5r43hV
6.1	Oocyte following ICSI showing second polar-body extrusion, pronuclear formation, and fading.	http://goo.gl/E2pkxp
7.1	Fragments arising at the two-cell stage and dispersed with subsequent cell divisions.	http://goo.gl/Uc5jSE
8.1	Development of a 3PN with 1PB.	http://goo.gl/h89nNE
9.1	Embryo compaction and blastulation.	http://goo.gl/yd3eJW
10.1	Blastocyst expansion and collapse.	http://goo.gl/Rarlz4
10.2	Morphokinetic time points in embryo development.	http://goo.gl/ibWDjn
11.1	A blastocyst expanding and then hatching through the zona pellucida.	http://goo.gl/y0zYFA
12.1	Embryo demonstrating multinucleation and irregular cleavage.	http://goo.gl/D3X0Xl
13.1	Irregular cell division and blastomere fusion.	http://goo.gl/rJMc5p
14.1	Large sERC in the oocyte cytoplasm.	http://goo.gl/8ujnQM
15.1	Blastomeres with multinuclei developing into an irregular cleavage pattern.	http://goo.gl/vi3EMT
16.1	Vacuoles developing in blastomeres at 60 hpi.	http://goo.gl/bS9bkJ
17.1	Granulation in the zygote cytoplasm and in the developing blastomeres.	http://goo.gl/Vi5Z2j
18.1	Development of an embryo with an atypical zona pellucida.	http://goo.gl/v3Upd7

1

Equipment Required for Time Lapse Observations in In Vitro Fertilization

Louise Best

Time-lapse imaging of human embryos has been used since the 1990s to study fertilization and early human embryo kinetics.[1] This early time-lapse cinematography collected images of inseminated oocytes every minute, for a period of 4 hours, using a low-light colour video camera positioned within a Perspex temporary incubation chamber on an inverted microscope using ×200 magnification which was augmented to ×1064 on a monitor. Technology has advanced since then to allow successive, noninvasive, interval imaging of an oocyte throughout the duration of the culture period from insemination onward in a culture dish without the need for it to be removed from its stable culture environment, until embryo transfer or cryopreservation.

Unlike the conventional single daily observations, time-lapse technology provides many hundreds of images and allows the marking of precise timings of key events in the embryo's development, prospective reviewing of the division patterns, and detection of brief but significant critical changes. These numerous images are linked by the software as a video of progressive embryo development over several days and displayed in just a few minutes. By archiving the performance of every embryo, a time-lapse database can be built. Images can be reannotated and data analyzed retrospectively in light of embryo fate and outcome.

The first live birth following time-lapse imaging of embryos was reported by Pribenszky and colleagues in 2010.[2] Since then, time-lapse imaging of embryos has rapidly become a key tool for clinical use and research in the field of human fertility.

Automated time-lapse observations in an in vitro fertilization (IVF) laboratory require images to be taken and recorded from a microscope while the culture dish remains within the incubated environment. The key elements of a time-lapse system are a high-resolution microscope; culture dish holding the embryo in such a way to reduce movement; software for capturing, analyzing, and recording the images; and the culture system. Several clinical time-lapse systems are commercially available for human clinical IVF practice. Each system differs in aspects of their design and operation. A key element of all of the systems is the manual or semiautomated interpretation of events and recording (or annotating) of the specific points in preimplantation development. These can either be system- or user-defined variables, but the software can then be used to calculate designated events, such as the time taken for an embryo to divide from one cleavage division to the next, or to annotate precisely the appearance or disappearance of defined structures. These annotations and calculations can then be used prospectively as

additional information in the choice of embryo, or embryos, for transfer or freezing.

Four different time-lapse systems, currently available at the time of print, are described in this chapter.

Primo Vision (Vitrolife, Sweden)

The Primo Vision Time-Lapse Embryo Monitoring System is a modular system that sits within a conventional IVF incubator and is connected to a controlling unit outside the incubator for continuous embryo monitoring (Figure 1.1). One unit is required for each patient. Dependent on the internal dimensions of the incubator, several Primo units can be placed within one incubator. The Primo Vision Evo is a compact digital inverted microscope that uses Hoffman contrast integrated optics with green LED (550 nm) illumination and can collect images through three to eleven focal planes.

The modular design allows expansion with additional microscopes to be installed at any time. The full system allows six microscopes to follow up to 96 embryos from six patients. The dishes are static below the camera for the duration of the culture time.

The Primo Vision embryo culture dishes are designed for this system and meet EU safety, health, and environment protection requirements (CE marked), are mouse embryo assay (MEA) tested, and are individually packaged (Figure 1.2). Depending on the patient requirements, dishes can hold up to 9 or 16 embryos of one patient in either three rows of three drops or four rows of four drops. The design of the dishes allows group culture while embryos are precisely identified and individually monitored within the 2.5 × 2.5 mm exposure area of the Primo Vision microscope. The dishes allow for use under normal stereomicroscope where embryos can also be identified if needed (Figure 1.2).

Primo Vision software captures, analyzes, and presents images for manual review. It provides a way to compare and analyze the development of embryos. Using the software, personalized reports and graphs can be created, and videos detailing embryo development can be shared with embryologists, clinicians, and patients. The system allows user-defined programming of the software to record morphokinetic variables and enables the precise observation of embryos' developmental dynamics from polar-body extrusion, pronucleus (PN) formation, through time points of cleavages and cleavage intervals. Notable events that can occur more than once can also be

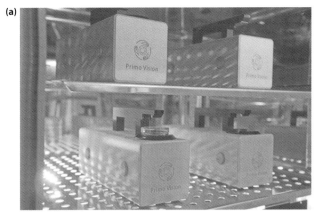

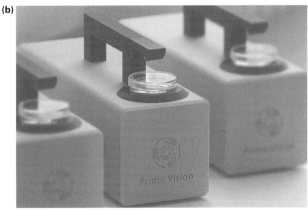

Figure 1.1 (a) Several Primo Vision EVOs set up inside a standard incubator. (b) Primo Vision Evo. (Courtesy of Vitrolife, Sweden.)

recorded for information including blastocoel pulsation and identification of fragmentation and cleavage patterns. It also allows published or in-house developed algorithms to be used to rank embryos accordingly in the 'compare function.'

A remote access feature allows access to the software imaging system from outside the laboratory. This means that embryos can be evaluated and assessed online by colleagues or other

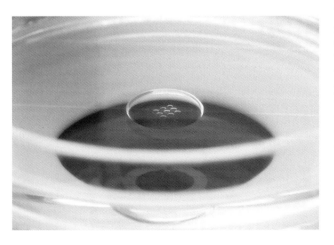

Figure 1.2 Primo Vision embryo culture dish. (Courtesy of Vitrolife, Sweden.)

professionals. The Primo Vision iPad Viewer allows viewing of the time-lapse images by IVF clinic professionals and patients.

As the Primo Vision Evo sits within an existing incubation system within a laboratory, this allows different culture conditions to be monitored, indeed different incubators, and so can provide a useful tool to maintain and improve overall lab quality. Measuring the effects on development of different culturing environments can be used to improve operating protocols by identifying when a negative factor is affecting results and tracking the root cause.

Eeva (Auxogyn, United States)

The Eeva (Early Embryo Viability Assessment) system is also a modular system that is housed inside a laboratory's existing conventional incubator (Figure 1.3). However, the system differs in the utilization of dark-field image capture, in a single focal plane, and automatic cell-division tracking. The system uses software to analyze early embryo development and provides quantitative data on each embryo's development potential to the blastocyst stage, based on the company's research into cell division timing parameters.[3]

Auxogyn's software, the Early Embryo Viability Assessment Test, aims to provide clinics and patients with objective information on embryo viability by giving an indication of each embryo's development potential to the blastocyst stage by tracking the progress for two days postfertilization. The Eeva scope fits into most standard IVF incubators and provides automatic dark-field image capture and cell-division tracking without intervention by the embryologist or excessive light exposure to the embryos. The quantitative, objective data, in conjunction with standard morphology grading, may enable IVF clinics to make better-informed decisions regarding embryo selection and the optimal patient treatment pathway at an early cleavage stage, on day 2. The Eeva test uses software that automatically analyzes embryo development against validated cell-division time periods and ensures objective measurements to assess embryo development when compared to manual methods (Figure 1.3). Auxogyn examined a wide range of potential noninvasive markers and gene expression data to assess embryo viability and proposes the greatest predictive power lies in the measure of time it took each embryo to achieve specific cell development milestones during the first two days after fertilization in vitro: (1) timing of the duration of first cytokinesis (i.e., the time from when the first cell division starts, to when it completes); (2) the time interval between cytokinesis 1 and cytokinesis 2 (i.e., the time from the two- to three-cell stage); and (3) the time interval between cytokinesis 2 and cytokinesis 3 (i.e., the time from the three- to four-cell stage).[3] This allows the transfer of embryos to take place on day 3 post insemination and eliminates the need for additional days in in vitro culture, with the associated risks including putative epigenetic effects.[4] The Eeva dish contains microwells that enable Eeva to track the individual development of up to nine embryos while allowing group culture technique. Using the Eeva station, images and videos for each Eeva patient session can be reviewed. The downloadable reports and videos may aid when counseling patients and improve the overall patient experience.

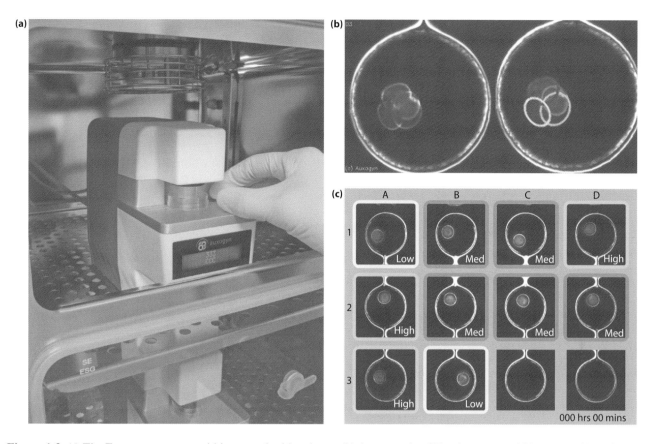

Figure 1.3 (a) The Eeva scope set up within a standard incubator. (b) An example of Eeva's automated blastomere identification feature, used to determine cell-division timing. (c) Eeva test results that display whether an embryo has a high, medium, or low development potential. (Courtesy of Auxogyn, USA.)

EmbryoScope (FertiliTech, Denmark)

The EmbryoScope is a stand-alone incubator/microscope unit that houses up to six patients in specialized slides. The incubator is nonhumidified with internal circulation of ultraviolet (UV)-light-sterilized air through a HEPA and volatile organic compound filtration system. It has an in-built red LED (635) illumination camera system that allows stable and uninterrupted time-lapse imaging. Dry incubation without water pans eliminates water condensation and associated fungal growth on surfaces (Figure 1.4).

The EmbryoScope can image up to 72 embryos, through a maximum of nine equidistant focal planes. This system includes embryo selection modeling software and provides tools for knowledge building through retrospective analysis of embryo development data.

The EmbryoScope utilizes an incubation slide that holds up to 12 embryos. Each embryo sits in 25 μL of media in a well with a central depression with a diameter of 0.2 mm. A vertical tail-fin on the slide ensures a firm grip and safe handling, and the lids have a small fin for easy detachment. Unique identification of each embryo is by means of a micronumeral next to the well bottom, visible through a dissection microscope. The EmbryoSlide tray fits perfectly into an instrument slide holder for direct heat transfer to media-filled wells. The water-impermeable polymer used to make the slide along with the cover of immersion oil prevent dehydration during handling in low-humidity laboratories and in dry incubators. The slides are individually packaged and are MEA toxicity tested and limulus ameobocyte lysate endotoxin tested (LAL). The EmbryoViewer Workstation allows the operator to review, annotate, and compare synchronized time-lapse movies of selected embryos. Multiple instruments can be connected to a single workstation, and embryos can be watched live from a remote location. The Zoi server supports secure data sharing within and between clinics using EmbryoScope. Patient data can be collected from multiple connected incubators and centralized in a common storage location.

Miri (Esco, Denmark)

The Esco Miri TL has six completely separate culture chambers, each taking 14 embryos with a total capacity of 84 embryos. Culture is in dishes called CultureCoins held in the individual chambers. Direct warming of the dishes in the chambers gives temperature stability and temperature recovery of 1 minute after door opening. Gas mixes ensure accurate control for the chambers, and the complete gas purge/exchange in the system leads to a gas recovery time of less than 3 minutes after door opening. Each compartment has a PT-1000 probe built in for temperature validation, and a pH sensor port is fitted as standard (Figure 1.5).

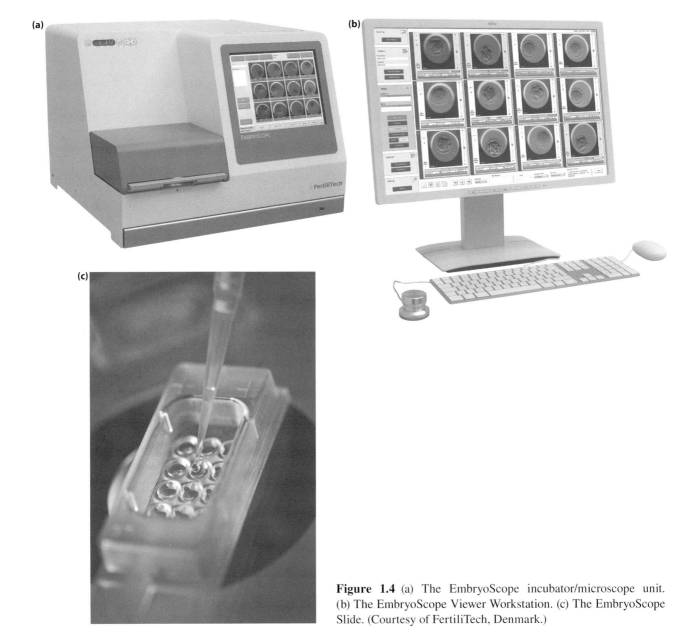

Figure 1.4 (a) The EmbryoScope incubator/microscope unit. (b) The EmbryoScope Viewer Workstation. (c) The EmbryoScope Slide. (Courtesy of FertiliTech, Denmark.)

Time-lapse monitoring uses multiple optical planes, with 5-minute picture intervals from throughout the culture period. User interaction is via a built-in high-definition (HD) resolution touch screen, with a large LED display adopting an event result–based drag-and-drop annotation.

To conclude, various alternative time-lapse systems are currently available for clinical use. With the increasing amount of supporting evidence for their use, this technology promises to bring opportunities for improved understanding of preimplantation embryo development and clinical outcome.[5-7] The key difference between the systems currently available is the requirement, or not, of existing IVF incubators. Image capture is performed using a camera system either placed into existing incubators (currently excluding bench-top-style low-volume incubators) or within an integrated incubator-imaging system.

Choice of device (Table 1.1) should be driven by the potential to impact positively on clinical outcome, opportunities for development and continuous improvement of the technology, device specification, focal planes, image quality and capacity, certification and licensing (where required), limitations, space, cost, customer support, servicing, and training.

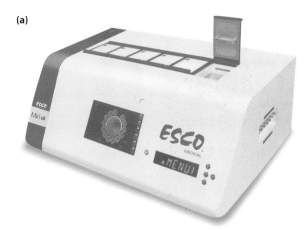

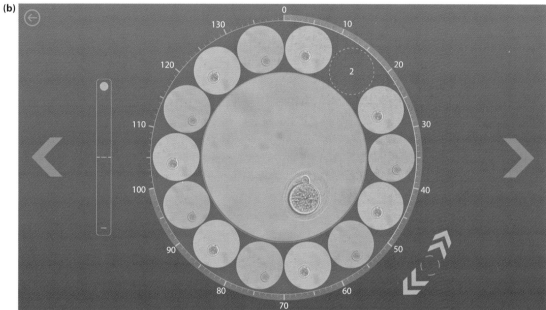

Figure 1.5 (a) (Image: Miri TL) The Esco Miri system. (b) CultureCoin. (Courtesy of Esco, Denmark.)

TABLE 1.1

Comparison of Time Lapse Systems Currently Available

	EmbryoScope	Eeva	Primo Vision	EscoMiri
Design	Stand-alone integrated incubator/microscope	Modular in standard incubator	Modular in standard incubator	Stand-alone integrated incubator/microscope
Maximum number of embryos monitored per dish	12	12	9 or 16	14
Single or group culture design	Single	Group	Group	Single
Total embryos in one system	72	48	54 or 96	84
Maximum number of focal planes	9	1	11	User defined No limit
Frequency of imaging	From 10 minutes (2 minutes with a single focal plane)	5 minutes	From 5 minutes	5 minutes
Imaging/illumination	Red LED	Dark field	Green LED	Red LED
Medical device registration	• CE Medical device Class IIa • FDA 510(k)	• CE and Canada approved • FDA submission pending	• System and dish both have CE marking	• CE Medical device Class IIa • FDA 510(k) pending

REFERENCES

1. Payne D, Flaherty SP, Barry MF, et al. Preliminary observations on polar body extrusion and pronuclear formation in human oocytes using time-lapse video cinematography. *Hum Reprod.* 1997;12:532–541.
2. Pribenszky C, Matyas S, Kovacs P, et al. Pregnancy achieved by transfer of a single blastocyst selected by time-lapse monitoring. *Reprod Biomed Online.* 2010;21:533–536.
3. Wong CC, Loewke KE, Bossert NL, et al. Non-invasive imaging of human embryos before embryonic genome activation predicts development to the blastocyst stage. *Nat Biotechnol.* 2010;28(10):1115–1121.
4. Shufaro Y, Laufer N. Epigenetic concerns in assisted reproduction: update and critical review of the current literature. *Fertil Steril.* 2013;99(3):605–606.
5. Meseguer M, Herrero J, Tejera A, et al. The use of morphokinetics as a predictor of embryo implantation. *Hum Reprod.* 2011;26(10):2658–2671.
6. Montag M, Toth B, Strowitzki T. New approaches to embryo selection. *Reprod Biomed Online.* 2013;27(5):539–546.
7. Campbell A, Fishel S, Duffy S, et al. Embryo selection model defined using morphokinetic data from human embryos to predict implantation and live birth. *ASRM.* 2013;24:P-1228.

2

Clinical Aspects of Time Lapse Imaging

Alison Campbell

Introduction

Morphological assessment of the preimplantation human embryo is the single and most commonly used method employed for embryo selection following IVF, and the correlation between embryo morphology and implantation potential has been extensively demonstrated and documented.

Typically, this morphological evaluation consists of up to six single, daily, conveniently scheduled observations during in vitro development to the blastocyst stage. Although, as stated, selection of the embryo(s) for transfer tends to be weighted toward the morphology of the embryo just prior to embryo transfer, other factors play a significant role. Assessing cell number at a particular time of development and the amount of fragmentation have led to simple embryo grading schemes, such as that utilized within the United Kingdom.[1] Other schemes include a more graduated approach to embryo scoring that takes into account several other variables such as pronuclear morphology.[2] More recently, the Istanbul consensus workshop on embryo assessment aimed to define common terminology and the minimum criteria for oocyte and embryo morphology assessment to allow effective comparisons and standardized reporting.

This published evidence-based grading scheme relies on morphological parameters as well as developmental stages being reached, each of which have been proven to be associated with embryo viability.[3,4]

Failure to select a viable embryo from a cohort will inevitably limit the chance of a positive outcome. The unwitting selection of a nonviable embryo, and the cryopreservation of viable alternative(s) within a cohort, will also delay the desired outcome. There is rapidly growing evidence to support that more emphasis should be given to the selection of embryos displaying optimal morphokinetic characteristics; however, assessment of morphokinetics (the morphology and dynamic behavior of the embryo, studied over time) is not possible when using standard incubation accompanied by static microscopical methods. The limited observations employed to minimize environmental stress to the embryos using this traditional 'snapshot' approach provide comparatively limited information on developmental rates or patterns.

The introduction of time-lapse microscopy as a clinical tool in IVF has resulted in several reports of improved embryo selection based on the analysis of sequential time-lapse images of embryo development. Time-lapse devices, now commercially available for the IVF laboratory, allow the capture of images of the embryos developing in vitro at regular intervals throughout the culture period. This provides continuous and uninterrupted monitoring that furnishes embryologists with a more sophisticated and promising tool for the study and selection of the human preimplantation embryo beyond conventional daily microscopy. The EmbryoScope was the first instrument to provide stable, uninterrupted incubation combined with internal microscopy. Meseguer et al., using this system, observed a 20 per cent increase in pregnancy rate compared to standard incubation and attributed this improvement to the EmbryoScope's stable culture conditions and use of morphokinetic variables for embryo selection.[5] Time-lapse technology also allows the identification of aberrant embryo cleavage that would not be observable using static traditional methods. An example of aberrant cleavage, which is reportedly common, is the phenomenon of a direct, or rapid, cleavage to three cells—in less than 5 hours.[6] This study demonstrated the ability of time lapse to identify aberrant cleavage divisions and highlights the reduced implantation potential when such embryos were transferred compared with embryos that did not exhibit this behavior. In a cohort of 1,659 transferred embryos, the incidence of this 'direct division' was 13.7 percent, and the known implantation rate of these embryos was markedly and statistically significantly lower than for embryos with a normal cleavage pattern (1.2 versus 20.2 percent, respectively). Importantly, this aberrant, but relatively common and clinically significant, cleavage had not been identifiable prior to time lapse being available.

There are multiple applications for time-lapse monitoring within the IVF laboratory. These include validation of conventional static assessment methodologies, prediction of embryo viability and outcome, comparison of the potential impact of variables such as culture media or drug regimens on morphokinetics, observation of transient or aberrant morphological phenomena, quality control, and improvement of flexibility and working patterns. This chapter considers practical aspects of time-lapse imaging, considers the use of morphokinetic data to develop embryo selection algorithms, and discusses how time lapse can be incorporated into the IVF laboratory in order to increase flexibility, information, and outcome for IVF patients.

Selection and Deselection Morphokinetic Criteria

Time-lapse monitoring of the dynamics of embryo development, in addition to traditional qualitative morphological observations, provides morphokinetic information on individual embryos. These data, generated by the manual or automatic recording (annotation) of the images, collected over precise time points, can be retrospectively analyzed against outcome variables, such as blastulation implantation, ploidy, or live birth. This type of analysis may allow practitioners to identify prospective and preferential selection criteria for embryo transfer or cryopreservation.

It is also effective in identifying exclusion, or 'deselection' criteria. For example, if a morphokinetic variable or event is shown to be associated with very poor clinical outcome, or even preclude implantation, embryos exhibiting this can be deselected for transfer, irrespective of their traditional morphological score.

Data Handling

Morphokinetic data from time-lapse monitoring systems should be precisely grouped according to known outcome following embryo transfer, for comparison and statistical analysis. Specific attention is required to exclude data following multiple embryo transfer that resulted in a lower number of fetal hearts or babies born than the number of embryos transferred. Additionally, inclusion of double embryo transfer morphokinetic data where two implantations resulted may be problematic without the use of genetic fingerprinting to ascertain the chorionicity or zygosity of the pregnancies. Due to the ranges observed for each morphokinetic variable, it is recommended that median values be used for comparison between successful and unsuccessful groups of embryos as opposed to means in order to avoid skewing the results. Once key significant variables have been identified, depending on the power of the data set available, they can be ranked according to their association with outcome and simple embryo selection algorithms, or models, developed.

Embryo Selection Algorithms

IVF clinics already use evidence-based biomarkers of embryo quality to aid their decision as to which embryo should be transferred or cryopreserved (e.g., early cleavage to two cells, presence of smooth endoplasmic reticulum aggregates), but this practice has limitations based on the static nature of the observation and often transient nature of the markers. Nevertheless, the embryologist may elect to use these existing selection or deselection criteria while building experience and data with a newly introduced time-lapse system, and while their individual, specific criterion is fine-tuned over time. For example, rather than using the current consensus value of 25 ± 1 hour, postinsemination, for early cleavage observation on day 1, as defined by the embryo grading and assessment guidelines, a more precise time point for this event, perhaps incorporating the insemination method, or patient factors, will in time be established for

that setting which relates to outcome.[3,4] It may then be incorporated into an embryo selection model.

The first morphokinetic-based model, which used specific timings to predict embryos most likely to develop to the blastocyst stage, was reported by Wong and colleagues in 2010.[7] Since then, prediction of blastulation, as a measure of embryo quality, or viability, has now been superseded by more robust clinical outcome measures such as ploidy, implantation, and live birth.[8-14]

Meseguer and colleagues used a hierarchical approach to modeling such that embryos received a classification based primarily on developmental milestones and relative timings associated with them. In a retrospective analysis of over 500 transferred embryos, where specific implantation data were available for 247, they found significant differences between implanted and not implanted embryos for six early morphokinetic variables, the most significant for implantation prediction being the time the embryo reached the five-cell stage (t5) and the duration of the second cell cycle (cc2). Their published model included three exclusion criteria based on their negative association with implantation. These were direct cleavage from one to three blastomeres, uneven blastomeres, and multinucleation at the four-cell stage.[8] More recently, Campbell and colleagues considered whether there was a difference in the morphokinetics of euploid and aneuploid embryos using data from blastocysts that had undergone biopsy and preimplantation genetic screening (PGS).[9] The only significant variables identified, from more than 20 variables compared, were the time to start blastulation (tSB) and the time to reach the full blastocyst stage (tB) defined according to their annotation system. From this, using recursive partitioning, they presented a risk classification model for aneuploidy.[9] More recently, Basile and coworkers have proposed a logistic regression–based model to improve the chance of selecting a euploid embryo from a cohort, based on morphokinetic data from embryos that underwent blastomere biopsy and PGS. They reported that chromosomally normal and abnormal embryos have different kinetic behavior and based the model on the significant morphokinetic variables t5-t2 and cell cycle three (cc3 = t5-t3).[15] Even though euploidy is crucial for optimum live birth outcome, there are clearly many more factors required within the embryo itself, and maternally, in order to ensure viability. For this reason, healthy live birth, rather than ploidy, is the ultimate outcome measure. Live birth was used as an outcome measure in a multiplicative model for early cleavage embryo selection. In this model, key variables and timings or intervals were weighted in order to create a ranking of embryos based on their predicted live birth potential. When morphokinetic profiles were compared between embryos that resulted in live birth and those that did not, the significant morphokinetic variables identified related to the first cleavage and early cell cycle lengths. Although a small study, this model is promising and was demonstrated to be very predictive of live birth as measured by the area under the receiver operating characteristic (ROC) curve (value was 0.8).[14]

Despite a number of morphokinetic embryo selection models now being published, it should be noted that such models may not be directly transferrable to another clinical setting. Inability of a model to be effectively reproduced in an alternative setting may be due to confounding factors, such as culture environment. For example, partial pressures of incubation gases or media used have been reported to influence morphokinetics, as have patient factors such as age and body mass.[16-18] It was recently demonstrated that the multivariate hierarchical selection model described above was not transferable from one clinical setting to another without modifications.[19] Conversely, the aneuploidy risk classification model, also referred to above, was effectively tested on large and independent data in relation to implantation outcome.[20] Whether pre-embryonic genome activation events, such as cleavage morphokinetics prior to the eight-cell stage, or later morphokinetic information representing the activated embryonic genome will give the most reliable selection criteria needs further study. Most published work to date has focused on events up to the five-cell stage, and as a prognosticator for blastulation, or implantation, rather than live birth.[7,8] While it is recognized that maternal effects may mitigate against the survival of the viable embryo, in any event—and not least because aneuploidy is the largest single cause of failure—live birth outcome, in relation to morphokinetics as a selection tool, should be the gold standard measure. While arguably easier, and consequently more objectively interpreted for annotation, they may not be as reliably representative of onward embryo development and potential following activation of the embryonic genome.

Need for Consensus

Consensus guidelines for professionals working with time-lapse monitoring in IVF do not exist currently, although with training workshops and forums often facilitated by device suppliers, there are opportunities for embryologists and researchers to compare and debate best practice. With an inevitably increasing proportion of IVF cycles now being conducted using time-lapse imaging, the need for professional guidelines for definition, interpretation, and annotation of images becomes a priority. Annotations are the records of morphological and dynamic events that provide the basis on which individual embryos can be evaluated and selected using defined criteria. Consistency in annotation, within the clinic, and the field will allow alignment of effective morphokinetic embryo evaluation.

The process of reaching proposed consensus for morphokinetic embryo selection, and acceptance of it, will be challenging due to the already existent heterogeneity within the published time-lapse studies and the lack of prospective randomized controlled trials to fully support the concepts. Many clinics experience difficulty in recruiting patients into these studies; this classical measure of 'evidence-based' data may delay consensus for morphokinetic embryo selection. However, these would be facilitated hugely by consensus guidelines for the annotation of time-lapse images and the definitions used to describe morphokinetic variables.

Second Opinions and Training

One of the key advantages of time-lapse systems in the IVF laboratory is the facility to allow clinical embryologists to rewind, pause, and review photographic frames in order to consider the detail and context of embryo development with practical flexibility without interruption of embryo culture. The storage of images also allows them to be reviewed retrospectively in order to reannotate further detail and perhaps consider novel events that went unrecorded previously (as noted in this atlas). It may be particularly worthwhile to annotate additional variables, for example, for embryos with known outcomes only. This would provide clinical relevance and possibility in the search for morphokinetic biomarkers for live birth outcome.

Quality Control and Assurance

As with many aspects of the embryologist's role, there are practical and efficiency benefits if multiple individuals are trained and competent in routine daily tasks. Time-lapse annotation is no exception, and once introduced into the laboratory, review, annotation, and interpretation of time-lapse images is currently considered a daily task. Where there are multiple practitioners involved, the risk of subjectivity and inconsistency is highest, although intrapractitioner annotation variation may also exist. Ensuring the most accurate and objective record of dynamic, often anomalous, embryo development brings challenges whether using automatic detection software or solo or collective manual methods. In order to minimize subjectivity, it is recommended that key variables for annotation be defined within the standard operating procedure (SOP) and that these be routinely recorded. With the current lack of consensus, policy should be set in house, adhered to, monitored, and refined where required. Core morphokinetic variables should be identified and annotated following rigorous training and competency assessment. Some morphokinetic variables are more at risk of subjective interpretation than others (e.g., the appearance of pronuclei). The use of reference images may be beneficial in assuring annotation quality.

The most commonly recorded morphokinetic variables follow the basic principles of embryology and mitosis and include timing of pronuclear appearance and fading, increasing cell numbers (time to two, three, four, five, six cells, etc.), and times of embryo differentiation to the morula and blastocyst stages. Durations of mitotic cycles and synchronicity can then be calculated from these. In addition, specific anomalies or phenomena associated can be annotated, depending on the customizability of the time-lapse system available.

Once established, a regular audit of annotation completion and quality and adherence to SOP is essential in order to maintain high quality data to allow analysis and opportunity for identification of significant selection or deselection morphokinetic criteria.

Early indications are that many of the morphokinetic events are recorded objectively, but it is critical that regular review and assessment exercises should be undertaken to assure quality. A study by Sundvall and colleagues considered inter- and intrapractitioner variation in annotation, using the intraclass correlation coefficient.[21] Their study demonstrated a close correlation between both experienced and new time-lapse users for most morphokinetic variables but highlighted that some 'static morphologic parameters' such as multinucleation and blastomere evenness remained at risk of subjectivity. With ongoing assessment and clear definitions and SOP, this can be minimized. Another report also found close correlation between annotators but highlighted how one misannotation could skew the data output.[22] In summary, until we know the potential impact of subtle deviations from protocol, culture dishes or slides should be prepared in a standard and precise fashion, and annotation of time-lapse images, where performed manually, performed with objectivity by all practitioners.

Flexibility and Opportunity

Due to the great interest in time-lapse technology by professionals in the field of IVF, the promising clinical results, opportunities to broaden knowledge of the preimplantation embryo's development, and its visual nature which appeals to clinic staff and patients, swift advances in the technology and the application of it are inevitable.

Computer servers, rather than stand-alone devices, will allow the support of new applications such as patient interface, improved data collection, storage, sharing, and remote access.

The Zoi server (FertiliTech, Denmark) is such a platform that supports secure data sharing within and between clinics using EmbryoScope. Patient data can be collected from multiple connected incubators and centralized in a common storage location. This enables IVF practitioners to view, annotate, and select embryos remotely which opens up new opportunities for productivity and flexibility. Before too long, time-lapse users may also expect statistical software packages for quality assurance and detailed analysis of data with associated embryo selection model building.

Summary

Within this rapidly progressing and promising area of reproductive medicine, practitioners now have an additional and increasingly reliable tool for improving embryo selection. It is yet unclear as to which patients may benefit most from this new approach, and reported significant uplifts in pregnancy and live birth rates by the use of this technology are still to be proven in large, randomized, controlled trials. However, it makes sense to observe and interpret the dynamic process of preimplantation embryo development, using technology that allows the dynamics to be studied, rather than a rigid and static, snapshot method, not least for the anomalies that can be excluded. The more we interrogate the collated images and data output, the more we can understand whether an optimal morphokinetic profile exists. The technology has the potential to provide embryo selection algorithms such that numerous criteria will be defined for a range of varying circumstances, from individual patient criteria to generalized laboratory conditions. In time, the optimal ranges for defined dynamic events such as those directly associated with the 'normal' cell cycle may be fine-tuned and further novel morphokinetic markers of embryo viability identified.

Time-lapse monitoring is a tool that not only dramatically increases flexibility in the IVF clinic but also has the potential to train, educate, and most importantly enhance clinical outcome.

ACKNOWLEDGMENTS

Many thanks go to Louise Kellam for her invaluable assistance and to CARE Fertility colleagues for their continued support and enthusiasm.

REFERENCES

1. Cutting R, Morroll D, Roberts SA, et al. Elective single embryo transfer for practice. British Fertility Society and Association of Clinical Embryologists. *Hum Fertil.* 2008;11(3):131–146.
2. Fisch J, Rodriguez H, Ross R, et al. The graduated embryo score predicts blastocyst formation and pregnancy rate from cleavage stage embryos. *Hum Reprod.* 2001;16:1970–1975.
3. Alpha Scientists in Reproductive Medicine and ESHRE Special Interest Group of Embryology. The Istanbul consensus workshop on embryo assessment: proceedings of an expert meeting. *Hum Reprod.* 2011;26(6):1270–1283.
4. Alpha Scientists in Reproductive Medicine and ESHRE Special Interest Group of Embryology. The Istanbul consensus workshop on embryo assessment: proceedings of an expert meeting. *Reprod BioMed Online.* 2011;22(6):632–646.
5. Meseguer M, Rubio I, Cruz M, et al. Embryo incubation and selection in a time-lapse monitoring system improves pregnancy outcome compared with a standard incubator: a retrospective cohort study. *Fertil Steril.* 2012;98(6):1481–1489.
6. Rubio I, Kuhlmann R, Agerholm I, et al. Limited implantation success of direct-cleaved human zygotes: a time-lapse study. *Fertil Steril.* 2012;98(6):1458–1463.
7. Wong CC, Loewke KE, Bossert NL, et al. Non-invasive imaging of human embryos before embryonic genome activation predicts development to the blastocyst stage. *Nat Biotechnol.* 2010;28(10):1115–1121.
8. Meseguer M, Herrero J, Tejera A, et al. The use of morphokinetics as a predictor of embryo implantation. *Hum Reprod.* 2011;26(10):2658–2671.
9. Campbell A, Fishel S, Bowman N, et al. Modelling a risk classification of aneuploidy in human embryos using non-invasive morphokinetics. *Reprod BioMed Online.* 2013;26(5):477–485.
10. Campbell A, Fishel S, Bowman N, et al. Retrospective analysis of outcome after using an aneuploidy risk model derived from time-lapse imaging without PGS. *Reprod Biomed Online.* 2013;27(10):140–146.
11. Herrero J, Alberto T, Ramsing NB, et al. Linking successful implantation with the exact timing of cell division events obtained by time-lapse system in the EmbryoScope. *Fertil Steril.* 2010;94(suppl 4):S149.
12. Cruz M, Perez-Cano I, Gadea B, et al. Time-lapse video analysis provides a correlation between early embryo division kinetics and subsequent blastocyst formation and quality. *Hum Reprod.* 2011;26:P-115.
13. Chamayou S, Patrizio P, Storaci G, et al. The use of morphokinetic parameters to select all embryos with full capacity to implant. *J Assist Reprod Genet.* 2013;30:703–710.
14. Campbell A, Fishel S, Duffy S, et al. Embryo selection model defined using morphokinetic data from human embryos to predict implantation and live birth. *ASRM* 2013;24 P-1228.
15. Basile N, Nogales MdC, Bronet F, et al. Increasing the probability of selecting chromosomally normal embryos by time-lapse morphokinetics analysis. *Fertil Steril.* 2014;101(3):699–704.

16. Leibenthron J, Montag M, Koster M, et al. Influence of age and AMH on early embryo development realised by time-lapse imaging. *Hum Reprod.* 2012;27:P-135.

17. Bellver J, Mifsud A, Grau N, et al. Similar morphokinetic patterns in embryos derived from obese and normoweight infertile women: a time-lapse study. *Hum Reprod.* 2013;28(3):794–800.

18. Ciray HN, Aksoy T, Goktas C, et al. Time-lapse evaluation of human embryo development in single versus sequential culture media—a sibling oocyte study. *J Assist Reprod Genet.* 2012;29(9):891–900.

19. Best L, Campbell A, Duffy S, et al. Does one model fit all? Testing a published embryo selection algorithm on independent time-lapse data. *Hum Reprod.* 2013;28(suppl 1):i87–i90.

20. Campbell A, Fishel S, Laegdsmand M. Aneuploidy is a key causal factor of delays in blastulation: author response to "A cautionary note against aneuploidy risk assessment using time-lapse imaging." *Reprod Biomed Online.* 2014;28(3):279–283.

21. Sundvall L, Ingerslev H, Knudsen U, et al. Inter and intra-observer variability of time-lapse annotations. *Hum Reprod.* 2013;28(suppl 1):i87–i90.

22. Murphy L, Hulme D, Jenner L, et al. Development of a quality assurance system for time lapse annotation. Poster presentation. Association of Clinical Embryologists conference, Sheffield, 2014.

3

Time Lapse, the Cell Cycle, Distribution of Morphokinetic Timings, and Known Implantation Data

Alison Campbell

Cell Cycles and Time Lapse Monitoring

A cell cycle is a series of complex events involving cellular and nuclear processes through particular phases that ensure the cell's division into two daughter cells. Mitosis consists of nuclear division and cytokinesis and consists of several phases: prophase, prometaphase, metaphase, anaphase, and telophase. These are preceded by interphase which encompasses stages GAP-1 (G1), Synthesis (S), and GAP-2 (G2) of what is known as the cell cycle. The duration of cell cycles in the human preimplantation embryo appears to be related to embryo viability.[1] Prolonged or rapid cell cycles could be associated with DNA repair, cellular rearrangements, or failure of an embryo to undergo cell cycle checkpoints. Both cycles could potentially compromise embryo development.[2]

The first cell cycle following fertilization has recently been described in detail following a large time-lapse study by Aguilar and colleagues.[3] In their study, they described initiation of the first cell cycle as the time from the completion of the second polar-body extrusion. The length of the S-phase (DNA replication) was defined as the time from appearance to the fading of two pronuclei. In this study, embryos with prolonged S-phase demonstrated significantly reduced implantation rates compared with embryos with S-phases ranging from 5.7 to 13.8 hours. Completion of the first cell cycle can be defined as the time point at which the embryo reaches the two-cell stage, such that the two daughter cells are discrete from each other.

Postinterphase cleavages of corresponding sister blastomeres rarely occur at precisely the same time, and so time-lapse users may also consider the synchronization of cell divisions within a round of mitosis, particularly as this has been reported to be correlated to embryo viability. The optimal value for this being reported is less than 0.76 hours.[4] This can be calculated by the synchrony of sister cell divisions. For example, synchrony of the second cell cycle would be defined as the duration of the transition of an embryo from two cells to four cells and is calculated by subtracting the time the embryo reached the three-cell stage (t3) from the time it reached the four-cell stage (t4). With frequent time-lapse image acquisition (such as every minute), the duration of each cytokinesis can also be measured from the time a cleavage furrow is first visible to the time that the daughter blastomeres are discrete from each other.[5]

Cell cycle duration is calculated using time-lapse annotation either according to a single cell division or as a round of mitosis whereby the number of blastomeres doubles. For the first cell cycle, as development begins with the single cell, these are the same. However, the second cell cycle begins with two cells, both of which should subsequently divide, forming two daughter cells each. There are therefore two individual blastomere cell cycles but a single embryo cell cycle, and this results in the doubling from two to four cells.

Figure 3.1 provides a schematic to represent the blastomere cell cycles (cc) and the rounds of divisions herein defined as embryo cell cycles (ECCs), resulting in the doubling from two to four and from four to eight cells. The cell cycle for blastomere a, is calculated as t3-t2 and documented as cc2a, and for blastomere b as t4-t2 and documented as cc2b. The cell cycle whereby the embryo reaches four cells from two cells (ECC2) is also calculated as t4-t2. The time that the last cleaving blastomere takes to cleave (from t2 to t4) equates to the duration of the ECC: All individual blastomeres cleave within this time frame. The same applies for the third cell cycle. The duration of the embryo's third cycle (ECC3) is the time it takes the embryo to develop from four to eight cells and includes four blastomere/cell cycles: a, b, c, and d. The cycle cc3a is t5-t4, cc3b is t6-t4, cc3c is t7-t4, and cc3d is t8-t4. Cycle ECC3 is t8-t4. The synchronization for ECC3 (S3) is calculated as t8-t5 as the period begins once the first of the four cells cleaves (Figure 3.1). Video 3.1 shows an oocyte post ICSI as it undergoes fertilization and cell division to a hatching blastocyst. The video pauses at the described morphokinetic time points; t0 is normally considered as the time at insemination (ICSI). The video can be viewed online: http://goo.gl/U6TN1n.

Morphokinetic markers depicted in Figure 3.1 and Video 3.1 are defined as follows, and unless otherwise stated, are considered as time post insemination (t0), generally recorded in hours; time to pronuclear fading (tPNf); time to two cells (t2), three cells (t3), four cells (t4), five cells (t5), and so forth; morula (tM); start of blastulation (tSB); and full blastocyst (tB).

Known Implantation Data (KID)

The precise timings or durations of an embryo's development, its pattern and movement (kinetics), alongside its morphology have

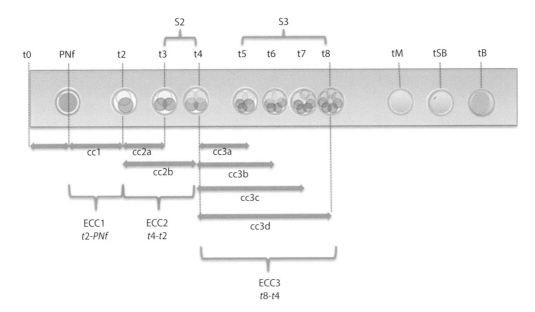

Figure 3.1 Three embryo cell cycles (ECC1, ECC2, and ECC3).

been referred to as its *morphokinetics*.[6] The morphokinetic data of a specific and transferred embryo which has a known outcome is commonly referred to as *known implantation data* (KID). The known outcome may be a pregnancy test result (positive or negative), a gestational sac or fetal heart on ultrasound scan, a pregnancy loss, or a live birth. Morphokinetic data can be compared between embryos giving positive or negative implantation data (KID+ or KID−), depending on the outcome measure used. All data can be utilized following a single embryo transfer, or a double embryo transfer with a negative outcome as the fate of these embryos is known. Using data, following multiple embryo transfer that has resulted in the same number of fetal hearts or babies born, may be problematic without the use of genetic fingerprinting to ascertain the chorionicity or zygoticity. However, in time, the level of monozygotic twinning can be established and factored to assess its significance and thereby the need for DNA fingerprinting.

Due to the ranges observed for each morphokinetic variable, it is recommended that median values are used as opposed to means. This way, extreme high or low values outliers do not introduce a skew.

The KID positive rates (or ratios) can be calculated for each morphokinetic variable in order to consider their impact and potential use in embryo selection models. Varied mathematical approaches, including recursive partitioning, have then been used in model development in order to ascertain significant and optimal time values, or ranges, for building embryo selection algorithms.[7]

Figure 3.2 shows a schematic representation of KID.

Distribution of Timings of Cleavages

These data represent over 9000 embryos (in vitro fertilization [IVF] and intracytoplasmic sperm injection [ICSI]) that underwent time-lapse monitoring at the CARE Fertility Group, United Kingdom, using EmbryoScope (FertiliTech, Denmark)

technology. The blue bars represent the numbers and morphokinetic timings for each variable of embryos which implanted, defined by the presence of a fetal heart on ultrasound scan (7 ± 1 week gestation). Timings are given in hours post insemination (hpi). Embryo culture was performed in microwells of 25 µL Global IVF medium (LifeGlobal®) supplemented with 10 percent Dextran serum supplement (Irvine Scientific), overlaid with 1.4 mL mineral oil (Fertipro, Belgium). Embryo culture took place at 37°C in 5.5 percent CO_2, 5 percent O_2, and 89.5 percent N_2. It is important to note that ranges of morphokinetic variables may vary according to gas tension, culture media, or patient factors, and clinics should consider their own data to establish expected ranges within their clinical practices.

The morphokinetic variables used in this evaluation are described within the text and in Figure 3.3. Durations of a distinct cell stage (or series of cell stages) can be obtained by subtracting one cleavage time from a later one (e.g., t7-t6 = duration of the six-cell stage).

Figure 3.3 shows a schematic representation of commonly used morphokinetic variables and calculated durations.

Time to Two Cells (t2)

The distribution of timings for the morphokinetic variable t2 in all embryos and in KID-positive embryos is shown in Figure 3.4.

Figure 3.4 supports the consensus based on static methodology that late t2 is associated with reduced implantation potential.[8] The upper limit for t2 in KID-positive embryos is 31 hpi; however, the majority of the embryos here were not transferred. Figure 3.4 also shows that first cleavage prior to 21 hpi is relatively uncommon at 1.2 percent of t2 data (*n* = 9,391) and that embryos that undergo this first cleavage prior to 21 hpi may have a lower incidence of known implantation compared to embryos with t2 in the 21 to 31 hpi range.

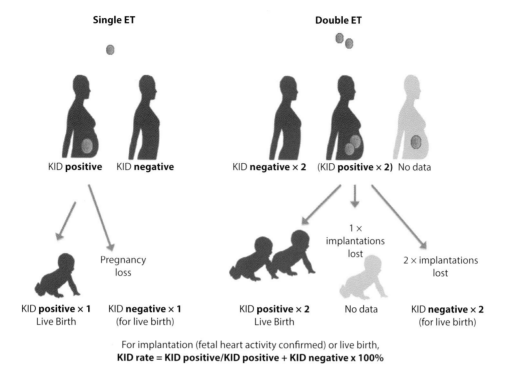

Figure 3.2 Schematic KID. (Modified from Alison Campbell, Non-invasive techniques: embryo selection by time-lapse imaging. In: Montag M, ed. *A Practical Guide to Selecting Gametes and Embryos*. Boca Raton, FL: CRC Press; 2014.)

Figure 3.4 shows a distinct range of t2 for preferential embryo selection and demonstrates how dynamic assessment of t2, as an example, provides practitioners with a tool that may allow the deselection, or exclusion, of embryos with t2 outside of a range that correlates to increased known implantation rates.

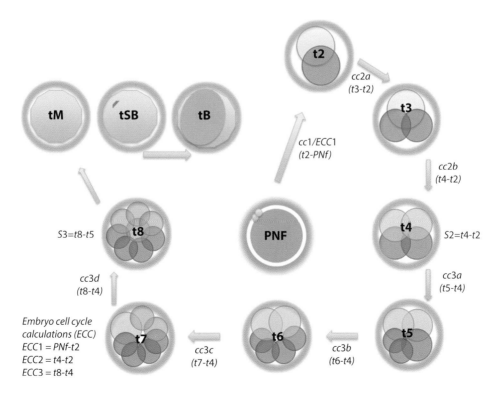

Figure 3.3 Morphokinetic variables.

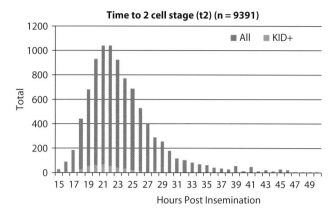

Figure 3.4 Distribution of timings for the morphokinetic variable t2 in all embryos and in KID-positive embryos.

Time to Three (t3) and Four (t4) Cells

The non-Gaussian distributions of timings for the morphokinetic variables t3 and t4 are shown in Figure 3.5. Optimal ranges for t3 and t4 are observed where the highest proportions of KID-positive embryos are present. These correspond, however, to the mode value for embryos overall.

Time to Five (t5) and Eight (t8) Cells

The non-Gaussian distribution of timings for the morphokinetic variables t5 and t8 are shown in Figure 3.6. The ranges for KID-positive embryos at t5 and t8 are broad, and the pattern of distribution, compared to embryos overall differs from those observed in Figure 3.5 for t3 and t4.

Time to Start Blastulation (tSB) and Time to Full Blastocyst Stage (tB)

The non-Gaussian distributions of timings for the morphokinetic variables tSB and tB are shown in Figure 3.7. For these variables, in contrast to the chronologically earlier variables discussed, the median values for tSB and tB in the KID-positive cohorts are earlier than the median values for the overall cohorts. These two morphokinetic variables were demonstrated to be delayed in preimplantation genetic screening (PGS)–confirmed aneuploid embryos compared with their euploid counterparts and have therefore been identified as potential morphokinetic variables for blastocyst selection models.[7]

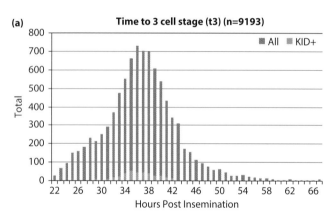

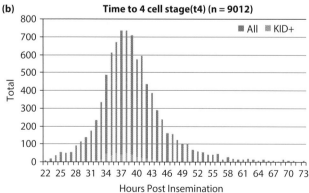

Figure 3.5 (a) Distribution of timings for the morphokinetic variable t3. (b) Distribution of timings for the morphokinetic variable t4.

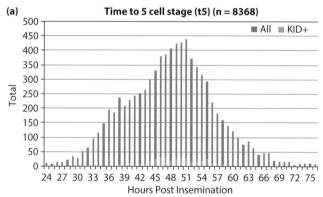

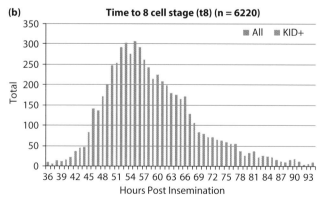

Figure 3.6 (a) Distribution of timings for the morphokinetic variable t5. (b) Distribution of timings for the morphokinetic variable t8.

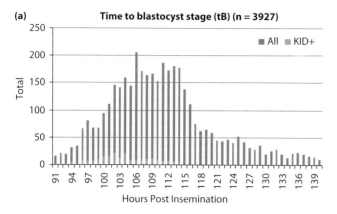

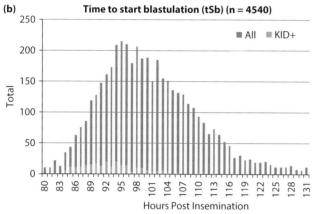

Figure 3.7 (a) Distribution of timings for the morphokinetic variable tSB. (b) Distribution of timings for the morphokinetic variable tB.

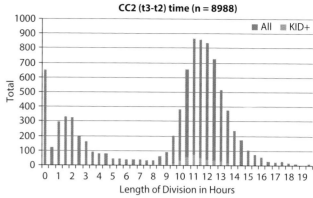

Figure 3.8 Second cell cycle (t3-t2) time (*n* = 8,988).

ACKNOWLEDGMENTS

With thanks to Louise Best for the preparation of the distribution figures.

Second Cell Cycle (cc2)

Time-lapse studies of rapid cleavage events to the three-cells stage (in less than 5 hours) have demonstrated this to be a morphokinetic criterion significantly associated with reduced implantation rates. Embryos displaying this irregular division pattern, described as *direct cleavage*, gave rise to implantation rates of 1.2 percent compared with 20.2 percent for embryos not displaying this division pattern.[8]

Analyses of the duration of the second cell cycle, in over 9000 embryos, at the CARE Fertility Group show a bimodal distribution with differing variance; the direct division from one to three cells (trichotomous mitosis), associated with the first peak, was less frequent than the division pattern when two cells were reached as an intermediate stage (Figure 3.8). The irregular division pattern in this cohort, represented by the first peak, is also associated with significantly reduced implantation.

This large analysis demonstrates that 26.3 percent of embryos undergo irregular cleavage, either directly (or rapidly) from one to three cells in less than 5 hours. Such events are not observable using static conventional assessment.

A peak for optimal cc2 range is observed where the highest number of KID-positive embryos are present (Figure 3.8).

REFERENCES

1. Ramsing NB, Callesen H. Detecting timing and duration of cell divisions by automatic image analysis may improve selection of viable embryos. *Fertil Steril.* 2006;86(suppl 3):S189.
2. Ramos L, de Boer P. The role of the oocyte in remodeling of the male chromatin and DNA repair: are events in the zygotic cell cycle of relevance to ART? *Biennial Rev Infertility.* 2011;2:227–243.
3. Aguilar J, Motato Y, Escribá MJ, et al. The human first cell cycle: impact on implantation. *Reprod Biomed Online* 2013;28:475–484.
4. Meseguer M, Herrero J, Tejera A, et al. The use of morphokinetics as a predictor of embryo implantation. *Hum Reprod.* 2011;26:2658–2671.
5. Wong C, Loewke KE, Bossert NL, et al. Non-invasive imaging of human embryos before embryonic genome activation predicts development to the blastocyst stage. *Nat Biotechnol.* 2010;28:1115–1124.
6. Meseguer M, Herrero J, Tejera A, et al. The use of morphokinetics as a predictor of embryo implantation. *Hum Reprod.* 2011;26(10):2658–2671.
7. Campbell A, Fishel S, Bowman N, et al. Modelling a risk classification of aneuploidy in human embryos using non-invasive morphokinetics. *Reprod Biomed Online.* 2013;26:477–485.
8. Rubio IR, Kuhlmann R, Agerholm I, et al. Limited implantation success of direct-cleaved human zygotes: a time-lapse study. *Fertil Steril.* 2012;98:1458–1463.
9. Alpha Scientists in Reproductive Medicine and ESHRE Special Interest Group of Embryology. The Istanbul consensus workshop on embryo assessment: proceedings of an expert meeting. *Hum Reprod.* 2011;26:1270–1283.
10. Alpha Scientists in Reproductive Medicine and ESHRE Special Interest Group of Embryology. The Istanbul consensus workshop on embryo assessment: proceedings of an expert meeting. *Reprod Biomed Online.* 2011;22:632–646.

4

Gender and Morphokinetics Correlation

Samantha Duffy

There are no studies published to date that comment on the relationship between embryos of known gender and their developmental patterns observed using time-lapse microscopy. Differences have been reported in conventionally assessed (static) morphology between male and female embryos suggesting that male embryos achieved full blastulation at a faster rate than did female embryos, and that a significantly higher proportion of male embryos were of a higher (morphological) grade than their female counterparts.[1]

CARE Fertility, an independent group of in vitro fertilization (IVF) centres in the United Kingdom, is conducting a study to establish whether embryo gender affects preimplantation embryonic developmental rates and patterns by retrospectively analyzing morphokinetic data obtained from the EmbryoScope (FertiliTech, Denmark). The first stage of this observational study included an analysis of results obtained from fresh intracytoplasmic sperm injection (ICSI) cycles that resulted in live birth. Eleven morphokinetic variables were studied for 43 embryos (19 female and 24 male) following 69 fresh ICSI cycles. Only embryos with a known implantation outcome were included in the study. The mean time points in hours post insemination (hpi) of the first cleavage (t2) up to the stage where embryos had greater than nine cells (t9+) and the time to reach morula (tM), full blastocyst (tB), and expanded blastocyst (tEB) were recorded for these embryos of known gender. (A complete explanation of morphokinetics values is presented in Chapter 2 (see Table 2.1)).

Although no statistical significance has been found to date with this sample size, the general trend observed for this cohort of embryos was for male embryos to develop at a faster rate up to eight cells and to full compaction (tM) but to blastulate and expand at a slower rate than female embryos.

The concept of differing morphokinetic values according to embryo gender is of scientific interest. The results of these preliminary analyses disagree with recent publications that have studied developmental patterns of known gender embryos cultured in standard incubation, with conventional observational practice that is limited by subjectivity and lacks precision compared with time-lapse imaging. The morphokinetic differences reported using time lapse between male and female embryos would be too subtle to be observed by static, single daily observation.

REFERENCE

1. Alfarawati S, Fragouli E, Colls P, et al. The relationship between blastocyst morphology, chromosomal abnormality and embryo gender. *Fertil Steril.* 2011;95(2):520–524.

5

Polar-Body Extrusion

Colleen Lynch and Mercedes Regueira

First polar-body extrusion occurs on completion of the first meiotic division of the oocyte, around the time of ovulation. As such this process is not normally observed via time-lapse imaging in the clinical setting. Following extrusion of the first polar body the second meiotic division commences, arresting at the metaphase 2 stage. Extrusion of the first polar body is taken as an indication of oocyte nuclear maturity and potential for fertilization (Figure 5.1).

The position of the first polar body is assumed to reflect the position of the maternal spindle, and so where intracytoplasmic sperm injection (ICSI) is performed, sperm is injected on a horizontal plane with the polar body at the 12 or 6 o'clock position. Injected metaphase 2 oocytes can be monitored using time-lapse image acquisition, with a device such as the EmbryoScope (FertiliTech, Denmark), and in those which fertilize normally, the extrusion of the second polar body will be observed. Extrusion of the second polar body is the first visible manifestation of fertilization and the conclusion of the second meiotic division. It cannot be taken as a definitive indication of normal fertilization as abnormally fertilized oocytes with one pronucleus (PN) may demonstrate extrusion of the second polar body (Figure 5.2). In abnormally ICSI-fertilized oocytes with three PNs, the second polar body is usually retained (Figure 5.3). Video 5.1 shows the development of a 3PN with 1PB. The video can be viewed online: http://goo.gl/ixaDhA.

Time-lapse imaging was first used to study and describe events of fertilization almost 20 years ago.[1] This preliminary observational study by Payne et al. described how normal fertilization followed a defined course of events and noted that the timing of the events described varied between oocytes. In the majority of fertilized oocytes (92 per cent), 'circular waves of granulation' within the ooplasm were observed. Extrusion of the second polar body and the formation of the second metaphase plate followed.

Using time lapse imaging in clinical practice allows the visualization of peri fertilization changes in the appearance of the cytoplasm. There is a brief contraction of organelles away from the cortex of the oocyte, accompanied by a glassy cytoplasmic appearance radiating out from the centre of the oocyte/cytoplasmic flare, which was described by Payne.[1] Video 5.2 shows second polar-body extrusion, cytoplasmic movements, and pronuclear formation and fading. The video can be viewed online: http://goo.gl/5r43hV.

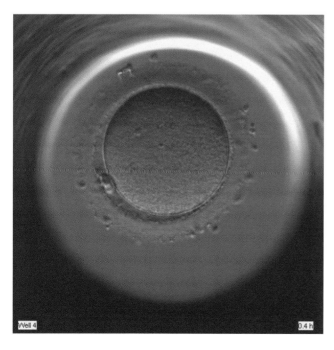

Figure 5.1 Metaphase II oocyte.

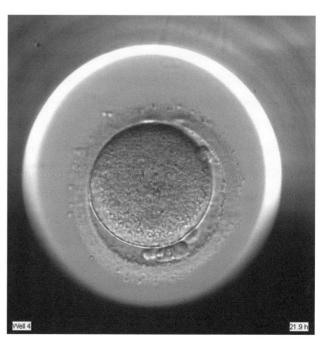

Figure 5.2 A single pronucleus and three polar bodies.

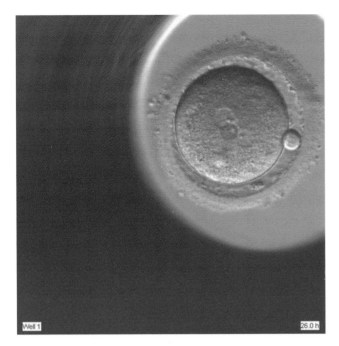

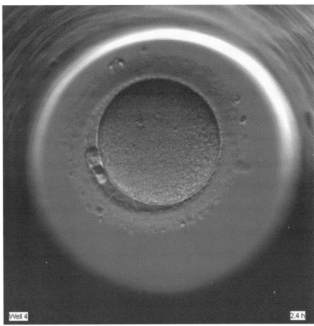

Figure 5.3 A tripronucleate zygote with single polar body.

Figure 5.4 Extruded polar bodies prior to PN formation.

Studies have shown a correlation between periodic cytoplasmic movements in mouse oocytes and development to the blastocyst stage.[2] These cytoplasmic rhythms, caused by contractions of the actomyosin cytoskeleton triggered by Ca^{2+} oscillations, are induced by fertilization. Human studies remain limited, but similar waves have been described in human oocytes but were not correlated to development.[3]

The female PN forms in the cytoplasm adjacent to the second polar body at the same time as or slightly after central formation of the male PN[1] (Video 5.2). The PN formation usually occurs within a few hours of second polar-body extrusion but is variable (Figures 5.4 and 5.5). The first polar body may divide during the second meiosis.

The second polar body is not always extruded adjacent to the first polar body (Figure 5.6). Displacement between the two can range from 0 to 180° and is observed in oocytes fertilized following ICSI and IVF.[1,4] Nonadjacent polar bodies indicate either spindle movement within the ooplasm or movement of the polar bodies within the perivitelline space. They also indicate that the location of the first polar body is not necessarily a reliable indicator of the location of the spindle. Additionally, movement of both polar bodies may be noted following extrusion (Figure 5.7).[5–7]

A number of studies indicate that timing of the extrusion of the second polar body is an indicator for embryo implantation and morphology. The second polar body may be extruded as early as 1 hour post ICSI, but extrusion less than 3.2 hours post insemination has been correlated with lower implantation rates.[8] A longer interval between ICSI and second polar-body extrusion has been linked to poorer embryo quality.[1] When looking at known implantation data, where the fate of a specific transferred embryo can be related to its morphokinetics, the optimal time for second polar-body extrusion was reported to

be 3.5 ± 1.43 hours following ICSI.[8] Looking at a larger data set, Aguilar established a range for second polar-body extrusion between 3.3 and 10.6 h post ICSI.[9]

A recent retrospective study at CARE Fertility of 310 transferred time-lapse monitored embryos with known outcome found that ICSI embryos with a greater distance between the polar bodies were significantly delayed in initiating blastulation (tSB) and reaching the full blastocyst stage (tB) compared with embryos

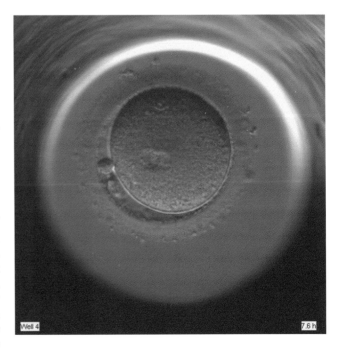

Figure 5.5 Extruded PBs and PN appearance.

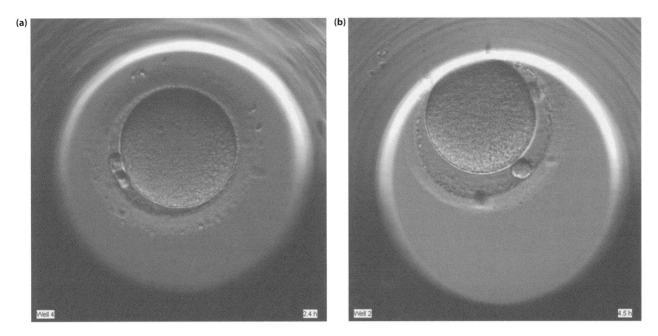

Figure 5.6 (a) Adjacent and (b) nonadjacent PBs.

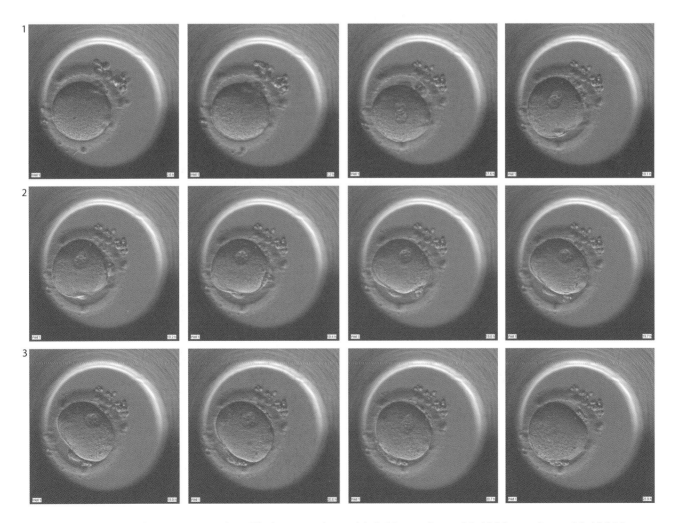

Figure 5.7 Movement of PBs post extrusion. (Timings: row 1, panel 1, 2.6 h; row 2, panel 1, 19.2 h; row 3, panel 1, 19.9 h.)

with adjacent polar bodies. These embryos also had significantly lower clinical pregnancy rates following blastocyst transfer.[10] As delayed tSB and tB were previously associated with the highest risk of aneuploidy, further work is required to establish whether PB2 alignment could be related with ploidy.[11] Moreover, it was observed that polar-body alignment is a time-dependent factor, and second polar-body relative position at a fixed time point is not a reliable reference to its position at extrusion.[10]

The morphology of the polar bodies can vary widely, from intact to completely fragmented, and have varying sizes. However, the majority of published data suggest this does not impact treatment outcomes.[12–14]

REFERENCES

1. Payne D, Flaherty SP, Barry MF, et al. Preliminary observations on polar body extrusion and pronuclear formation in human oocytes using time-lapse video cinematography. *Hum Reprod.* 1997;12:532–541.

2. Ajduk A, Ilozue T, Windsor S, et al. Rhythmic actomyosin-driven contractions induced by sperm entry predict mammalian embryo viability. *Nat Commun.* 2011;2:417.

3. Swann K, Windsor S, Campbell K, et al. Phospholipase C-ζ-induced Ca2+ oscillations cause coincident cytoplasmic movements in human oocytes that failed to fertilize after intracytoplasmic sperm injection. *Fertil Steril.* 2012;97:742–747.

4. Garello, Baker H, Rai J, Montgomery S, et al. Pronuclear orientation, polar body placement, and embryo quality after intracytoplasmic sperm injection and in-vitro fertilization: further evidence for polarity in human oocytes? *Hum Reprod.* 1999;14:2588–2595.

5. Cooke S, Tyler JP, Driscoll GL. Meiotic spindle location and identification and its effect on embryonic cleavage plane and early development. *Hum Reprod.* 2003;18:2397–2405.

6. Hardarson T, Lundin K, Hamberger L. The position of the metaphase II spindle cannot be predicted by the location of the first polar body in the human oocyte. *Hum Reprod.* 2000;15:1372–1376.

7. Rienzi L, Ubaldi F, Martinez F, et al. Relationship between meiotic spindle location with regard to the polar body position and oocyte developmental potential after ICSI. *Hum Reprod.* 2003;18(6):1289–1293.

8. Drew C, Hickman CF, Best L, et al. A time lapse investigation using the EmbryoScope (Unisence, Denmark) into the timing of PB2 extrusion to review the standard operating procedure for clinical preimplantation genetic screening (PGS). Association of Clinical Embryologists 8th Annual Conference, 2–4 January 2012, Leeds; P0025.

9. Aguilar J, Motato Y, Escribá MJ, et al. The human first cell cycle: impact on implantation. *Reprod Biomed Online.* 2014;28(4):475–484.

10. Reguiera M, Cater E, Jenner L, et al. Retrospective assessment of second polar body alignment using time lapse imaging. ESHRE Annual Conference, 29 June 2014, Milan P-093.

11. Campbell A, Fishel S, Bowman N, Duffy S, Sedler M, Hickman CF. Modelling a risk classification of aneuploidy in human embryos using non-invasive morphokinetics. *Reprod Biomed Online.* 2013;26:477–485.

12. Ciotti PM, Notarangelo L, Morselli-Labate AM, Felletti V, Porcu E, Venturoli S. First polar body morphology before ICSI is not related to embryo quality or pregnancy rate. *Hum Reprod.* 2004;19(10):2334–2339.

13. Di Berardino T, Chronis Brown P, Holt D, Nichols T, Greenblatt E. The morphology of the First Polar Body (1st PB) is not related to embryo quality and pregnancy rate after ICSI. *Fertil Steril.* 2006; 86(3):S320.

14. Yakin K, Balaban B, Isiklar A, Urman B. Oocyte dysmorphism is not associated with aneuploidy in the developing embryo. *Fertil Steril.* 2007; 88(4):811–816.

6

Fertilization: Pronuclear Formation and Fading

Louise Kellam and Laina Murphy

Observation of the presence and number of pronuclei is regarded as a reliable method of confirming fertilization. Observing the dynamic process of pronuclear formation and fading, however, has not been possible without time-lapse technology. Video 6.1 shows an oocyte following ICSI showing second polar-body extrusion, pronuclear formation, and fading. The video can be viewed online: http://goo.gl/E2pkxp.

In vivo and after conventional in vitro fertilization (IVF), corona and cumulus cells surrounding the oocyte make detailed continuous observations difficult at the point of spermatozoon-oocyte fusion and transition to zygote. However, with the use of intracytoplasmic sperm injection (ICSI) and time-lapse technology, it is now possible to study pronuclear formation and fading alongside other morphokinetic variables.

The appearance of two centrally positioned pronuclei within the oocyte cytoplasm, with clearly defined membranes and two polar bodies in the perivitelline space, indicates normal fertilization. The two pronuclei are haploid as a result of meiosis in both gametes. When only a single pronucleus or greater than two pronuclei are observed, fertilization is considered abnormal. These zygotes are therefore avoided for transfer in clinical IVF treatments as they are associated with a low viable pregnancy rate and a potentially abnormal fetus.[1] The phenomenon of abnormal zygotes is described in more detail later in this chapter.

Spermatozoon penetration of the arrested oocyte in the dictyate stage, in meiotic prophase, induces intracellular calcium oscillations that activate the fertilized oocyte to undergo the transition to zygote, involving major changes in the molecular signals that control the oocyte's arrest.[2] As a result, one set of chromatids are extruded in the second polar body. The set of chromatids remaining in the cytoplasm, localized near the point of emission of the second polar body, progressively form vesicles that group to form a visible female pronucleus. Meanwhile, the inactive and condensed spermatozoon nucleus decondenses and is transformed to a functioning male pronucleus within the oocyte cytoplasm. There are a number of overlapping stages to this transformation: removal of the spermatozoon nuclear envelope and disassembly of nuclear lamina; substitution of protamines with histones leading to initial chromatin decondensation and then recondensation; rebuilding of the nuclear envelope; rapid demethylation of spermatozoon DNA; and finally, swelling of the male pronucleus and its migration toward the female pronucleus.[3]

During pronuclear formation, nuclear precursor bodies can be visualized within the forming pronucleus. They migrate and merge into visible larger nucleoli (Figure 6.1). The nucleoli are considered to be extremely important, as this is where ribosomal RNA transcription and assembly take place and the embryonic genome becomes active. The nucleoli can be observed using time-lapse microscopy and continuously move and align along the edge of the nuclear envelope where the pronuclei juxtapose (Video 6.1). This alignment together with the morphology of the pronuclei has been suggested as being predicative of embryo competence.[4–6] However, there is inconclusive data on the clinical efficacy of single static pronuclear morphological evaluation, and some believe there is no value.[7] None of the tested pronuclei scoring systems to date have been demonstrated to predict the live birth outcome in a time-lapse setup.[8]

The male and female pronuclei can be seen drawing toward each other until they abut. Both increase in size, the nucleoli move around within the pronuclei, and some nucleoli coalesce. In the time-lapse study by Payne et al. (1997), using an image acquisition frequency of 1 minute during the fertilization period, they noted that oocytes decrease in diameter during pronuclear formation and that the female pronucleus is significantly smaller in diameter and contained fewer nucleoli than the male pronucleus. They also noted cytoplasmic waves of granular cytoplasm moving in a clockwise or anticlockwise direction just prior to the extrusion of the second polar body and formation of the male pronucleus.[9] Mouse studies have reported an association between cytoplasmic movements, or flows, in oocytes and blastocyst development.[2] These particular movements are caused by contractions of the actomyosin cytoskeleton triggered by calcium oscillations induced by fertilization. Similar flows have been identified in a human study on aged oocytes.[10] With less frequent image capture, this phenomenon may not be observed using clinical-use time-lapse systems, although textural cytoplasmic differences are observable (Video 6.1).

The spermatozoon's centrosome plays a leading role in the organization of the oocyte microtubules which directs the positioning of both pronuclei within the cytoplasm. As the male and female pronuclei abut, the centrosome is deposited between them and remains linked to the male pronucleus until syngamy.[4,18] Using confocal immunofluorescence microscopy, studies of the human oocyte have shown a specific pronuclear alignment associated with a polarized distribution of both male and female chromatin, along with the position of the sperm centrosome and the microtubules nucleating from it.[2] The extrusion of the second polar body sets the polar axis. Alignment of the two pronuclei on this axis is essential for the formation of polar

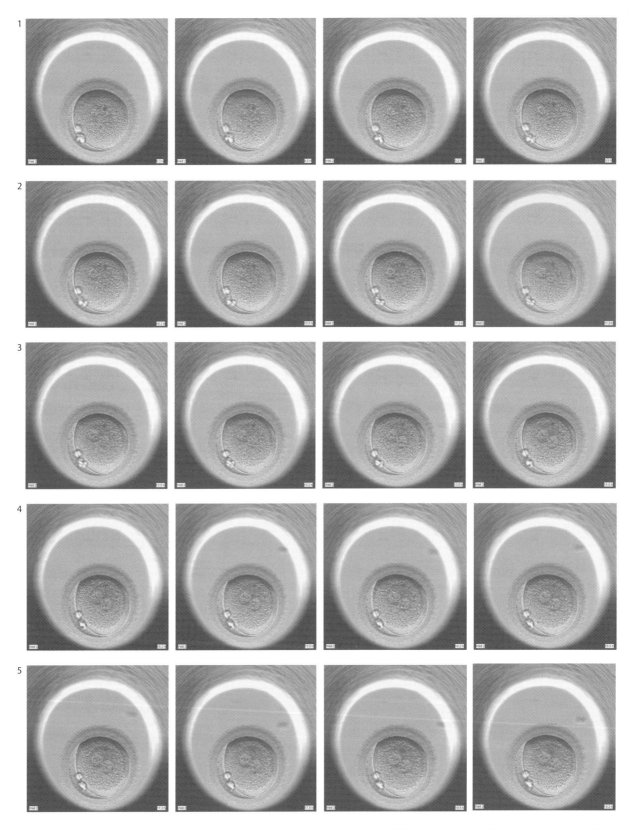

Figure 6.1 Series of time-lapse images showing the formation of the pronuclei, 0.2-hour intervals. The first image is at 8.2 hours post ICSI. By 10.2 hours, faint pronuclei can be seen, with the most peripheral likely to be the female pronucleus. By 12 hours, two nuclei are fully formed, and nucleoli clear. (Timings: row 1, panel 1, 68.2 h; row 2, panel 1, 10.2 h; row 3, panel 1, 12.5 h; row 4, panel 1, 15.2 h; row 5, panel 1, 17.2 h; row 6, panel 1, 19.9 h; row 7, panel 1, 22.2 h; row 8, panel 1, 24.5 h; row 9, panel 1, 27.2 h.)

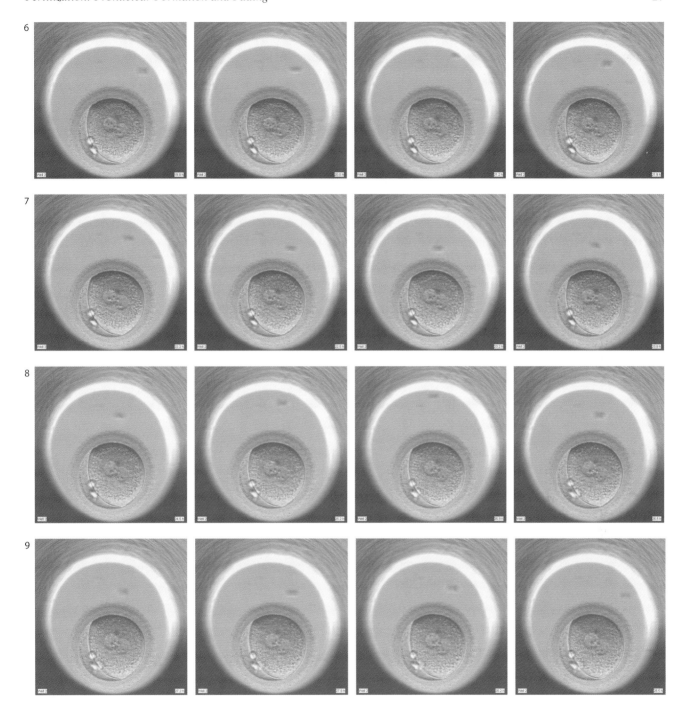

Figure 6.1 (Continued)

axes at syngamy and the subsequent plane of the first cleavage division and development.[9] When the two pronuclei are peripherally located, the pronuclear axis and subsequent cleavage plane may be disrupted, and cleavage may not occur regularly. Development of embryos arising from peripheral pronuclei is poor and arrest is likely; however, implantations have been reported.[4,11]

Pronuclear migration/juxtaposition to the centre of the oocyte is accompanied by the withdrawal of mitochondria and other organelles from the cytoplasm as they accumulate around the pronuclei. As a result, the peripheral cytoplasmic area is left relatively deprived of subcellular structures and appears translucent.[12] Commonly referred to as a *cytoplasmic halo*, this observation has been used as a predictor of embryo competency. However, current consensus is that there is insufficient evidence to support its prognostic value[6,13] (Figure 6.1).

Generally, both male and female pronuclei appear synchronously. An early study showed the time from ICSI to pronuclear formation varied between eggs but that they were morphologically similar at the end of the recording period. If one pronucleus did form before the other, it was always the male.

Formation was observed between 3 and 10 hours, with 50 percent forming by 5 hours post injection.[9]

Approximately 18 to 24 hours after spermatozoon fusion with the oolemma, the chromosomes in the pronuclei recondense, and the pronuclear membranes break down and are no longer visible, commonly referred to as *pronuclear fading*. Syngamy occurs, and the male and female chromosomes merge to form a diploid zygote. The two centrioles of the centrosome then migrate to opposite ends of the mitotic spindle to determine polarization. This allows the organization of the condensed chromosomes on the spindle for correct segregation and replication of the DNA during the first mitotic division. As the pronuclear membranes do not fuse, no membrane-bound, diploid nucleus is seen in the human zygote as in other species, such as the sea urchin. Instead the first visible diploid nuclei are observed at the two-cell stage.

The pronuclear fading is seen as a relatively sudden event, happening within the 6- to 12-minute image capture interval on a time-lapse recording (Video 6.1). As pronuclear fading is complete within a few minutes it is easy to annotate using time-lapse software. As a result, pronuclear fading may be selected as an objective start point in a laboratory's process to develop a morphokinetic embryo selection model, rather than time of insemination that cannot be easily defined on a per oocyte basis (Figure 6.2).

An in-house retrospective time-lapse study at CARE Fertility looked at the pronuclear fading dynamics of 1,192 embryos.[14] Data from embryos with positive known implantation were analyzed and compared to those that failed to implant. All transferred embryos that resulted in implantation demonstrated pronuclear fading between 16.5 and 30 hours post ICSI insemination. The embryos that failed to implant demonstrated a wider range of pronuclear fading between 16.5 and 50.35 hours, with 6 percent of embryos demonstrating pronuclear fading after 30 hours. This study suggests that late pronuclear fading may be associated with reduced implantation potential.

There is a commonly used window for fertilization check of 16 to 18 hours post insemination, as recommended by consensus guidelines.[13] Interestingly, in another time-lapse study at CARE Fertility, the presence of two pronuclei was observed at 18 hours post ICSI insemination in 91 percent of zygotes. However, 9 percent of the zygotes had pronuclei appearing after 18 hours and would have been missed had static traditional fertilization checks taken place at this particular time. Nevertheless, all zygotes with known implantation potential had two pronuclei visible at 18 hours.[15]

Using time-lapse imaging at CARE Fertility, dynamic pronuclear formation anomalies have been observed. Zygotes with dysmorphic pronuclei, and asynchronous fading of pronuclei have been recorded (Figures 6.3 and 6.4). As more time-lapse data are collected, our understanding of the significance of these anomalies will be enhanced.

With continuous monitoring there is no requirement for a fixed time window for a fertilization check. This allows flexibility with insemination timings and the opportunity to visualize morphokinetic events and anomalies that would otherwise have been overlooked with conventional observational methods. The accumulation of time-lapse recordings and annotations may help to establish a predictive value of pronucleus formation patterns and anomalies with respect to embryo competency, potentially leading to revised scoring systems in the future.[16,17]

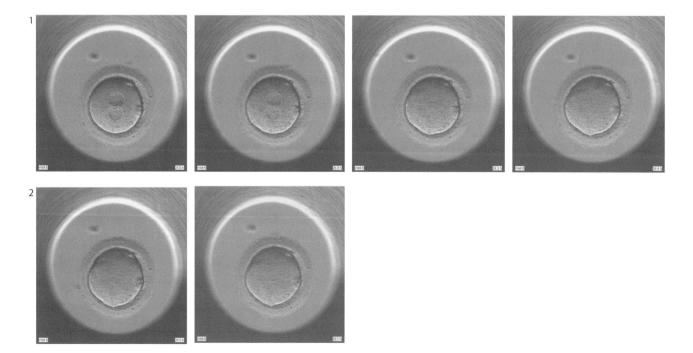

Figure 6.2 Series of time-lapse images showing pronuclear fading. At 25.9 hours (row 1, panel 1) the pronuclei are distinct, 6 minutes later (row 1, panel 2) they are visible yet less defined, and by 26.2 hours (12 minutes later, row 1, panel 3), they have both faded completely. (Timings: row 1, panel 1, 25.9 h; row 2, panel 1, 26.5 h.)

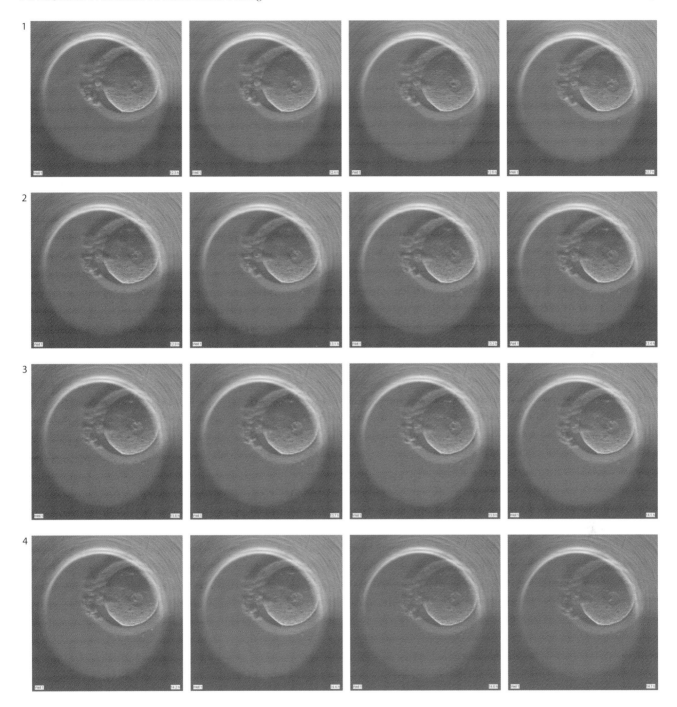

Figure 6.3 Series of time-lapse images showing dysmorphic pronuclei from 12.3 hpi (row 1, panel 1) to 14.4 hpi (row 4, panel 2), one presenting larger than the other. By 16.4 hpi the smaller pronucleus had faded, and at 26.4 hpi, the larger pronucleus faded. (Timings: row 1, panel 1, 12.3 h; row 2, panel 1, 12.9 h; row 3, panel 1, 13.6h; row 4, panel 1, 14.2 h.)

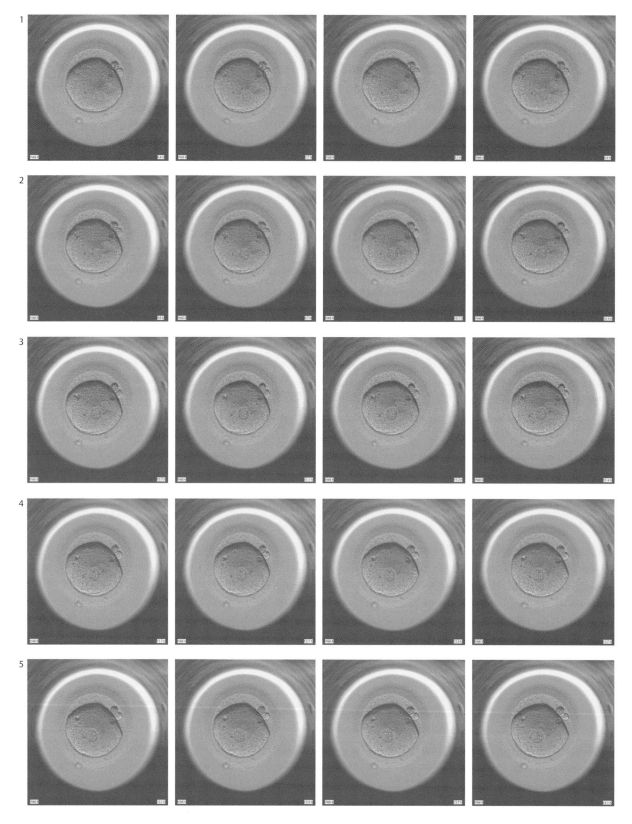

Figure 6.4 Series of time-lapse images showing asynchronous fading of pronuclei. Two even-sized nuclei and two polar bodies are seen clearly at 8.4 hours, indicating normal fertilization. By 11.6 hours one pronucleus begins to fade. By 16.4 hours only one pronucleus is clearly visible, with no visible sign of the second. The oocyte appears as a 1PN now, until the single remaining pronucleus fades at 19.1 hours. (Timings: row 1, panel 1, 8.4 h; row 2, panel 1, 9.6 h; row 3, panel 1, 10.7 h; row 4, panel 1, 11.7 h; row 5, panel 1, 13.1 h; row 6, panel 1, 14.4 h; row 7, panel 1, 15.4 h; row 8, panel 1, 16.4 h; row 9, panel 1, 17.7 h.)

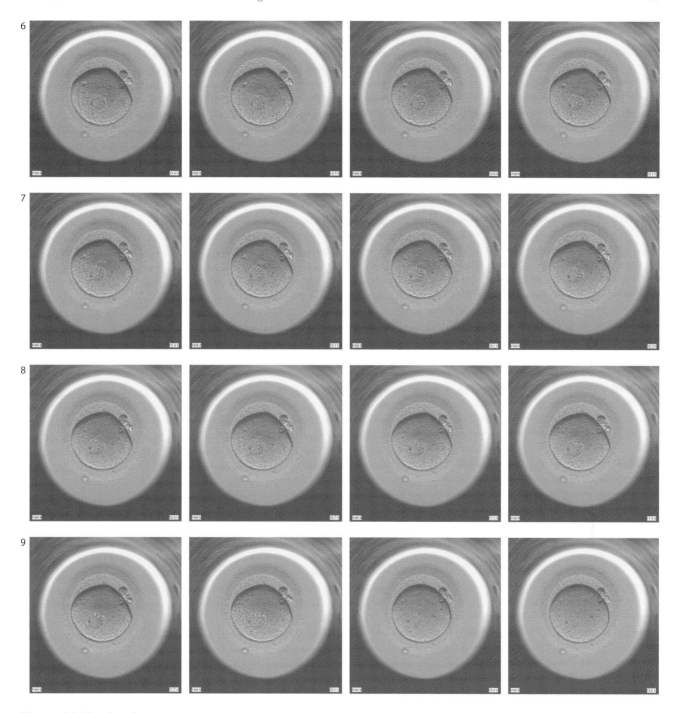

Figure 6.4 (Continued)

REFERENCES

1. Reichman DE, Jackson KV, Racowscky C. Incidence and development of zygotes exhibiting abnormal pronuclear disposition after identification of two pronuclei at the fertilization check. *Fertil Steril.* 2010;94:965–970.
2. Ajduk A, Ilozue T, Windsor S, et al. Rhythmic actomyosin-driven contractions induced by sperm entry predict mammalian embryo viability. *Nat Commun.* 2011;2:417.
3. Fulka H, Mrazek M, Tepla O, et al. DNA methylation pattern in human zygotes and developing embryos. *Reproduction.* 2004;128:703–708.
4. Scott L. Pronuclear scoring as a predictor of embryo development *Reprod Biomed Online.* 2003;Mar;6(2):201–214.
5. Tesarik J, Junca AM, Hazout A, et al. Embryos with high implantation potential after intracytoplasmic sperm injection can be recognized by a simple, non-invasive examination of pronuclear morphology. *Hum Reprod.* 2000;15:1396–1399.

6. Tesarik J, Greco E. The probability of abnormal preimplantation development can be predicted by a single static observation on pronuclear stage morphology. *Hum Reprod.* 1999;14:1318–1323.

7. Nicoli A, Palomba S, Capodanno F, et al. Pronuclear morphology evaluation for fresh in vitro fertilization (IVF) and intracytoplasmic sperm injection (ICSI) cycles: a systematic review. *J Ovarian Res.* 2013;6:64.

8. Azzarello A, Hoest T, Mikkelsen A, et al. The impact of pronuclei morphology and dynamicity on live birth outcome after time-lapse culture. *Hum Reprod.* 2012;27(9): 2649–2657.

9. Payne D, Flaherty SP, Barry MF, et al. Preliminary observations on polar body extrusion and pronuclear formation in human oocytes using time-lapse video cinematography. *Hum Reprod.* 1997;12:532–541.

10. Swann K, Windsor S, Campbell K, et al. Phospholipase C-ζ-induced Ca^{2+} oscillations cause coincident cytoplasmic movements in human oocytes that failed to fertilize after intracytoplasmic sperm injection. *Fertil Steril.* 2012;97:742–747.

11. Papale L, Fiorentino A, Montag M, et al. The zygote. *Hum Reprod.* 2012;27(suppl 1):i22–i49.

12. Coticchio G, Brambillasca F. The choreography of fertilization. In: Coticchio G, Albertini D, De Santis L, et al., eds. *Oogenesis.* New York, NY: Springer; 2012:300–301.

13. Alpha Scientists in Reproductive Medicine and ESHRE Special Interest Group of Embryology. The Istanbul consensus workshop on embryo assessment: proceedings of an expert meeting. *Hum Reprod.* 2011;26:1270–1283.

14. Sivanantham S, Nice L, Campbell A, et al. A comparative study on pronuclear fading timings and implantation using embryos cultured using time lapse imaging. *Fertility.* 2014. Published abstract.

15. Sivanantham S, Nice L, Campbell A, et al. Validation of pronuclear assessment timings using embryos cultured using time-lapse imaging. *Fertility.* 2014. Published abstract.

16. Montag M, Liebenthron J, Koster M. Which morphological scoring system is relevant in human embryo development? *Placenta.* 2011;32:S252–S256.

17. Herrero J, Meseguer M. Selection of high potential embryos using time-lapse imaging: the era of morphokinetics. *Fertil Steril.* 2013;99:1030–1034.

18. Sathananthan AH, Ratnam SS, Ng SC, et al. The sperm centriole: its inheritance, replication and perpetuation in early human embryos. *Hum Reprod.* 1996;11(2):345–356.

7

Clinical Results: Dynamic Aspects – Fragmentation

Sue Montgomery

Fragmentation is a common feature of human embryo cleavage stage development in clinical in vitro fertilization (IVF) programmes, but its etiology is poorly understood. It has been shown to occur in human embryos grown in vivo and so does not appear to be exclusively due to in vitro culture conditions.[1,2] Various mechanisms have been suggested, such as an apoptotic process, helping to rid the embryo of cells that are not viable, but not all evidence supports this theory.[3] The viability of human fragmented embryos is extremely difficult to predict, as many fragmented embryos are known to be developmentally competent and can produce live births, but it is generally recognized that this is to a lesser extent than their unfragmented counterparts.[4]

Fragmentation has been shown to be related to reduced viability and blastocyst formation rates, when more than 15

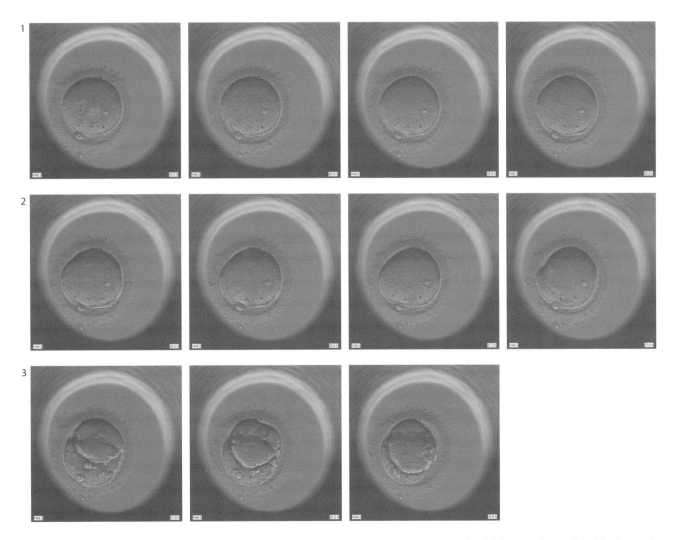

Figure 7.1 Fragmentation usually arises at the first cleavage division. (Timings: row 1, panel 1, 25.2 h; row 2, panel 1, 26.5 h; row 3, panel 1, 27.9 h.)

percent fragmentation occurs at the cleavage stage.[5,6] It is currently not possible to distinguish in a cohort of fragmented embryos, which embryos are capable of implanting. It is possible that the release of large fragments at the cleavage stage may deplete the embryo of essential organelles, such as mitochondria (essential for normal cleavage) or polarized membrane constituents.[4] However, it has also been suggested that this may vary according to the pattern of fragmentation.[7] In Alikani's categorization, scattered large fragments that were indistinguishable from cells were specifically associated with a significantly lower blastocyst formation rate.

Fragmentation may interfere with the compaction process, affecting cell-to-cell contact as intracellular junctions form between blastomeres. Any blastomeres or cellular fragments that are unable to form contacts with other cells are usually excluded from the compaction process and hence from further embryo development.

Time lapse information demonstrates that usually fragmentation arises at the first cleavage division, as the embryo cleaves to the two-cell stage. Video 7.1 shows fragments arising at the two-cell stage and dispersed with subsequent cell divisions. The video can be viewed online: http://goo.gl/Uc5jSE. It is rare for it to begin at the second or third cleavage division, when the embryo is progressing to the three- or four-cell stage (Figure 7.1).[8]

Patterns of fragmentation have been described previously, as localized to one area of the embryo (Figure 7.2), or dispersed.

However, the use of time lapse demonstrates that the fragments can change from being localized in one area of the embryo and scattered between the cells and back again, with subsequent cleavage divisions. There is no known link to outcome associated with this.

During the process of compaction, fragments can be either totally included (Figure 7.3) or partially excluded (Figure 7.4) from the compaction process.

A recent study has demonstrated that embryos displaying fragmentation at the cleavage stage are able to produce euploid blastocysts, both when fragments are excluded from compaction and when they are included.[8] Interestingly, there was a relationship between the duration of compaction time and the ploidy status of the resultant blastocyst, from fragmented embryos, with significantly more euploid blastocyst reported when compaction was completed within 22 hours.[8]

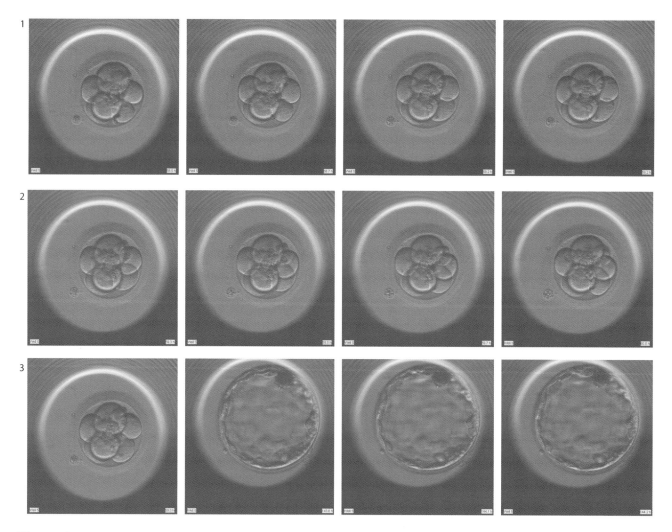

Figure 7.2 Fragments can be localized to one area of the embryo. (Timings: row 1, panel 1, 58.5 h; row 2, panel 1, 59.3 h; row 3, panel 1, 59.0 h.)

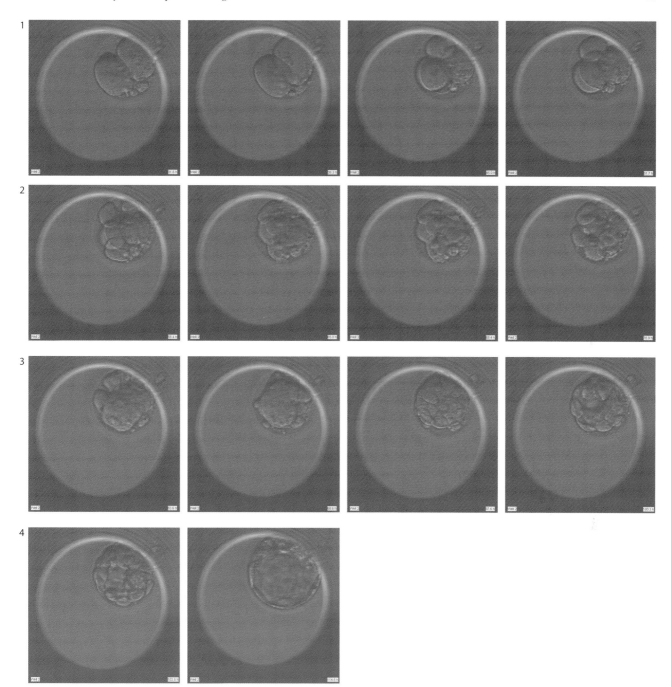

Figure 7.3 Fragments can be included at the compaction stage in embryos that progress to full blastocysts. (Timings: row 1, panel 1, 31.6 h; row 2, panel 1, 58.4 h; row 3, panel 1, 83.6 h; row 4, panel 1, 102.6 h.)

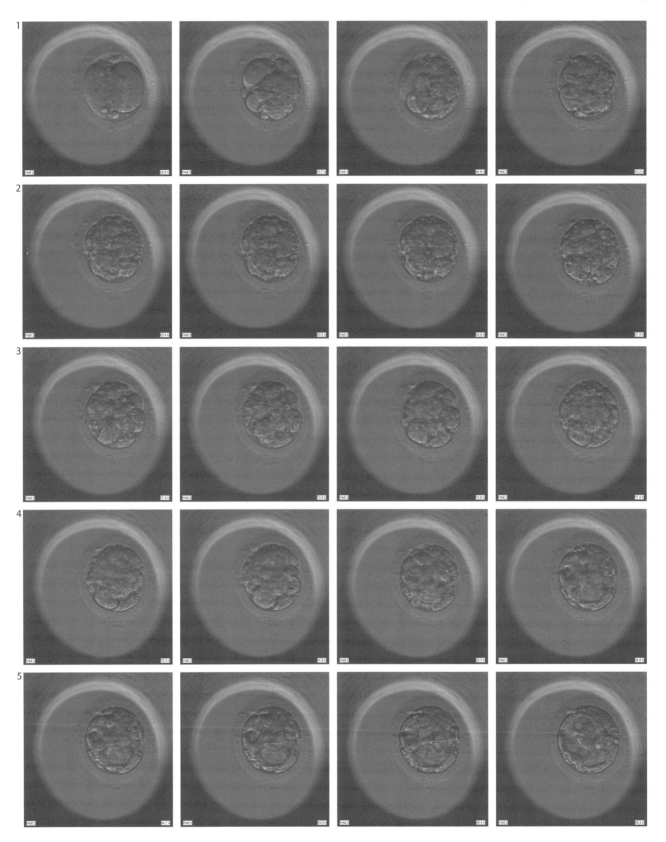

Figure 7.4 Fragments can be excluded at the compaction stage in embryos that progress to full blastocysts. (Timings: row 1, panel 1, 29.9 h; row 2, panel 1, 58.4 h; row 3, panel 1, 71.9 h; row 4, panel 1, 79.3 h; row 5, panel 1, 94.7 h; row 6, panel 1, 99.7 h; row 7, panel 1, 101.9 h; row 8, panel 1, 102.5 h; row 9, panel 1, 109.7 h.)

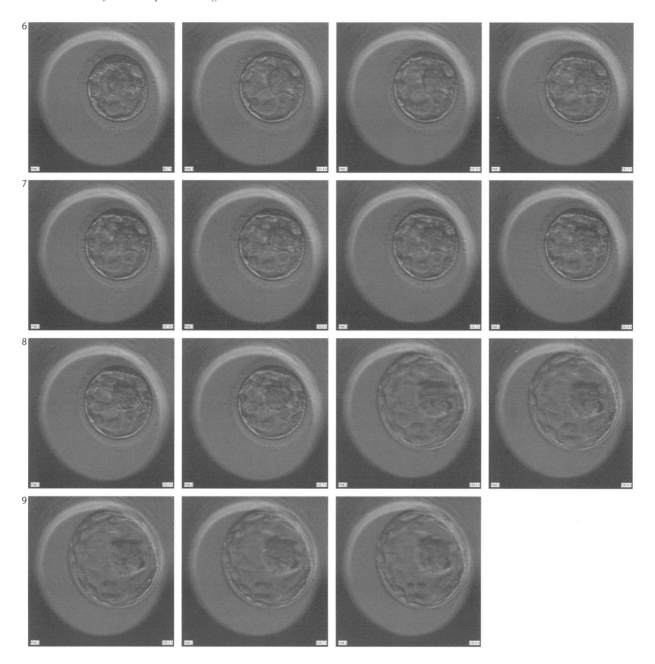

Figure 7.4 (Continued)

REFERENCES

1. Pereda S, Cheviakoff S, Croxatto HB. Ultrastructure of a 4-cell human embryo developed in vivo. *Hum Reprod.* 1989; 4:680–688.

2. Formigli L, Roccio C, Belotti G, Stangalini A, Coglitore MT, Formigli G. Non-surgical flushing of the uterus for pre-implantation recovery: possible clinical applications. *Hum Reprod.* 1990;5:329–335.

3. Levy R, Benchaib M, Souchier C, Guerin JF. Annexin V labelling and terminal transferase-mediated DNA end labelling (TUNEL) assay in human arrested embryos. *Mol Hum Reprod.* 1998;8:775–783.

4. Antczak M, Van Blerkom J. Temporal and spatial aspects of fragmentation in early human embryos: possible effects on developmental competence and association with the differential elimination of regulatory proteins from polarized domains. *Hum Reprod.* 1999;14:429–447.

5. Giorgetti C, Terriou P, Auquier P, et al. Embryo score to predict implantation after in-vitro fertilisation: based on 957 single embryo transfers. *Hum Reprod.* 1990;10:2427–2431.

6. Alikani M, Cohen J, Tomkin G, Garrisi J, Mack C, Scott RT. Human embryo fragmentation in vitro and its implications for pregnancy and implantation. *Fertil Steril.* 1999;71: 836–842.

7. Alikani M, Cohen J. Patterns of cell fragmentation in the human embryo in vitro. *J Assist Reprod Genet.* 1995;12:28S.

8. Montgomery S, Duffy S, Bowman N, et al. Does the duration of compaction differ in embryos that become euploid or aneuploid blastocysts? *Hum Reprod.* 2013;28:i1–i4.

8

Number of Pronuclei and Ploidy in IVF/ICSI–Derived Embryos

Abigail A. Burchill

Following insemination, an oocyte may form different numbers of distinct pronuclei, with anything other than two (with two polar bodies also present) being an indication of possible abnormal fertilization. These zygotes have the potential to develop and implant; however, they can be associated with pregnancy abnormalities. It is therefore important in the assisted reproductive technology (ART) setting to identify such anomalies and avoid transferring the resulting embryos into the uterus.

Unipronucleate (1PN) fertilization occurs at a rate of approximately 2 to 5 percent of all inseminated oocytes in ART cycles with approximately 9 percent reported following intracytoplasmic sperm injection (ICSI) and 3 percent after in vitro fertilization (IVF).[1–4]

The 1PN zygotes can form by parthenogenesis, and will be haploid, or more commonly as a result of either premature pronuclear fusion or asynchronous pronucleus formation, and will be diploid (46 to 80 percent). These diploid zygotes can be identified in time-lapse culture as the dynamics of pronuclear appearance and merging are observable along with polar-body extrusion events that may be missed during standard fertilization checks. To accurately determine the type of 1PN present and ascertain whether a zygote has normally fertilized, some authors have utilized fluorescent in situ hybridization (FISH) techniques to look for the presence of a Y chromosome.[2–5] Figure 8.1 illustrates an oocyte inseminated by ICSI which extrudes the second polar body at 2.1 hours post insemination (hpi) but appears to be unipronucleate.

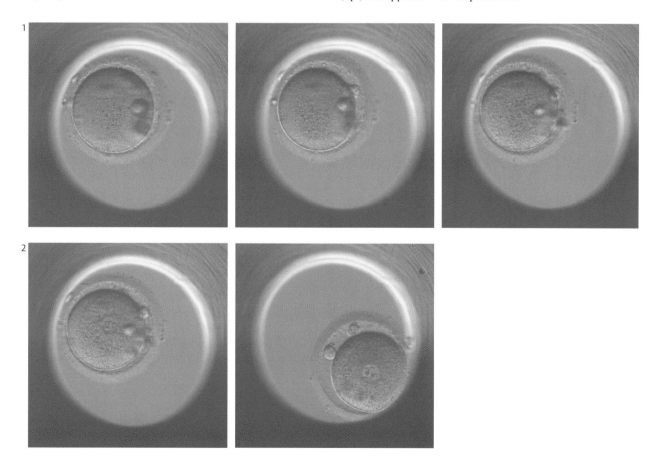

Figure 8.1 An oocyte extruding the second polar body at 2.1 hpi but appearing to be unipronucleate. (Timings: row 1, left to right: 0.1–9.1 hpi; row 2, left to right: 12.3–19.4 hpi.)

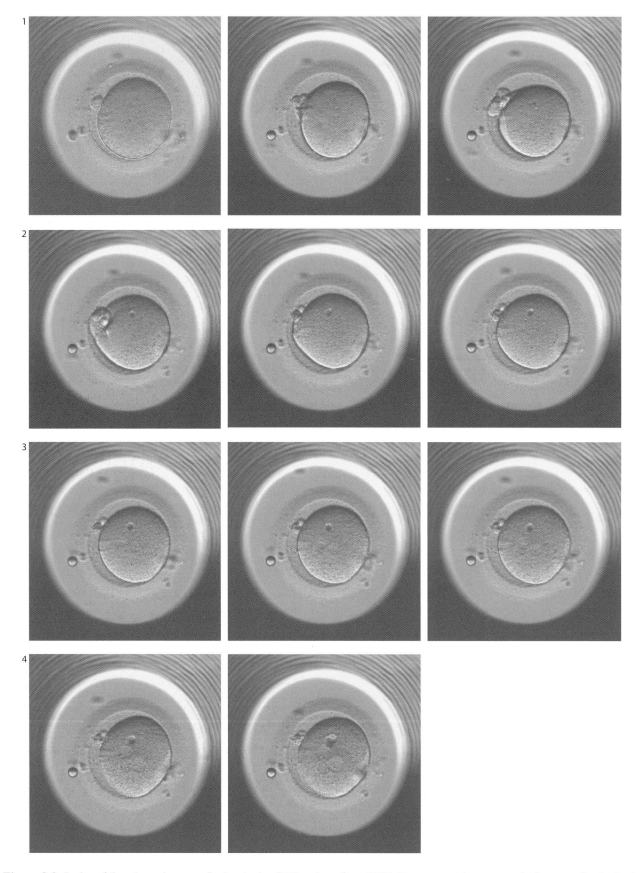

Figure 8.2 Series of time-lapse images of a developing 3PN embryo from ICSI. The oocyte tries to extrude the second polar body at 3.2 to 4.9 hpi position but fails to completely, resulting in a triploid zygote (digynic). (Timings: row 1, left to right: 0.3–3.7 hpi; row 2, left to right: 4.4–5.2 hpi; row 3, left to right: 6.4–7.9 hpi; row 4, left to right: 10.4–13.1 hpi.)

A study by Levron et al. looked at 1PN zygotes from IVF using FISH and found that out of 16 analyzed, 6 were diploid, 4 of which had XY chromosomes (therefore, they must have been fertilized by a sperm) and 2 had XX chromosomes.[6] As no DNA was detected in the cytoplasm, they postulated that the production of diploid (fertilized) 1PN oocytes in IVF will be mainly due to fused pronuclei and not asynchronous appearance of the pronuclei. The remaining 10 zygotes were haploid (and no DNA was present in the cytoplasm); therefore, these must have been produced by parthenogenesis.[5] Most ICSI 1PNs are due to parthenogenesis and are not diploid (only 9.5 percent of ICSI 1PN's were diploid), but in IVF, most (61.6 percent) were diploid and approximately half of these had a Y chromosome suggesting normal fertilization by a haploid sperm.[3,4]

Polyploid fertilization in human IVF/ICSI usually consists of 3PN (triploidy) (Figure 8.2), 4PN (tetraploidy), and rarely >4PN zygotes (Figure 8.3). Video 8.1 shows the development of a 3PN with 1PB. The video can be viewed online: http://goo.gl/h89nNE. Polyploidy is also a relatively common occurrence in human ART, particularly in IVF cycles, occurring in approximately 5 percent of inseminated oocytes.[6] The resulting embryos will theoretically carry more than the required two sets of homologous chromosomes in each cell. Triploidy (3PN), in particular, is a common cause of pregnancy abnormalities, accounting for approximately 15 to 18 percent of aborted pregnancies.[1] If implanted, triploid embryos usually lead to miscarriages, blighted ova, and partial hydatidiform moles. Accounting for around 1 in 10 000 live births, if born, these babies usually die soon after birth due to multiple congenital abnormalities.[1,7] See Figure 8.2 for time-lapse images of a digynic triploid zygote.

The most common cause of triploidy is diandric fertilization due to the oocyte being deficient in activating the block to polyspermy and allowing two spermatozoa to penetrate the oolemma. In ICSI, only 1 percent of zygotes will be polyploid and arise by fertilization by a diploid spermatozoa or, more commonly, the failure of the egg to extrude the second polar body. This digynic fertilization is the result of a failed meiotic division during oogenesis, producing a diploid oocyte or following fertilization by a single spermatozoa and a failure to extrude a polar body from the oocyte.[2,6] Digynic-fertilized oocytes usually survive longer in utero or neonatally than diandric embryos, although diandric embryos are more common and ultimately they will all be lethal.[7]

Abnormal fertilization is reportedly increased in oocytes fertilized by ICSI where the meiotic spindle is ≥90° in relation to the polar body leading to failure of extrusion of the second polar body.[8] The polar body can be displaced in relation to the

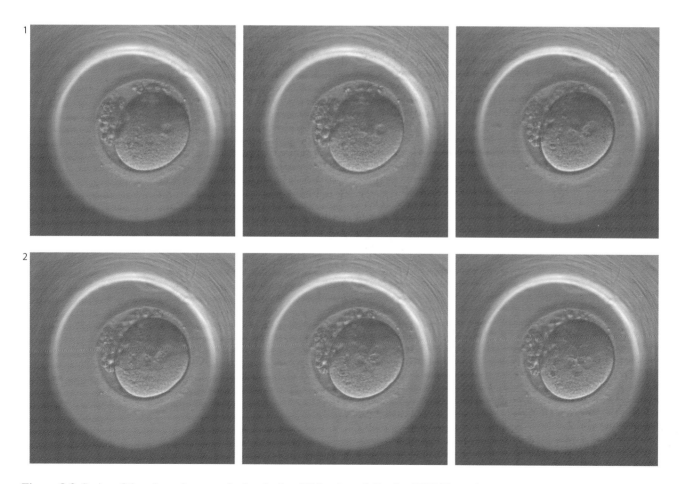

Figure 8.3 Series of time-lapse images of a developing 5PN embryo following ICSI illustrating pronuclei appearing. Embryo was 2PN at 18.6 hpi and four PNs were visible by 21.9 hpi, and then a fifth PN developed subsequently. Crucially, this anomaly may have been missed if time lapse were not used. (Timings: row 1, left to right: 18.6–21.9 hpi; row 2, left to right: 23.2–26.4 hpi.)

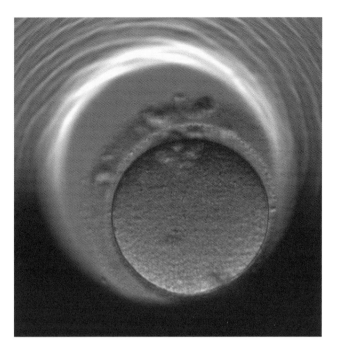

Figure 8.4 Giant unfertilized MII oocyte.

oocyte during mechanical stress of denudation of cumulus and coronal cells; therefore, mechanical stresses need to be avoided to reduce abnormal fertilization.[8]

Other contributors to digyny are 'giant' oocytes (Figure 8.4). Giant oocytes (with ≥30 percent increase in cell volume) occur at a rate of approximately 0.3 percent in ART.[7,9] Giant oocytes will usually be diploid, and these should not be inseminated as they often lead to triploid, tetraploid, or mosaic embryos. They can consist of either one or two metaphase plates (with 46/2 × 23 sets of chromosomes, respectively). When fertilized, giant oocytes can appear normal (have 2PN) but one pronucleus can be diploid, therefore making the zygote polyploid. These abnormal zygotes can cleave and blastulate normally, too, despite their abnormal cytogenetic makeup; therefore, it has been suggested that giant oocytes/embryos are not utilized. Giant oocytes are linked to high estradiol levels and excessive follicular response and are produced by abnormal cell division during mitosis of oogonia or fusions of oogonia during development.[7,9]

REFERENCES

1. Figueira RCS, Setti AS, Braga AS, et al. Prognostic value of triploid zygotes on intracytoplasmic sperm injection outcomes. *J Assist Reprod Genet.* 2011 September; 28(10):879–883.
2. Munne S, Cohen J. Chromosome abnormalities in human embryos. *Hum Reprod Update.* 1998;4(6):842–855.
3. Staessen C, Van Steirteghem AC. The chromosomal constitution of embryos developing from abnormally fertilized oocytes after intracytoplasmic sperm injection and conventional in-vitro fertilization. *Hum Reprod.* 1997;12(2):321–327.
4. Sultan KM, Munné S, Palermo GD, et al. Chromosomal status of uni-pronuclear human zygotes following in-vitro fertilization and intracytoplasmic sperm injection. *Hum Reprod.* 1995;10(1):132–136.
5. Levron J, Munne S, Willadsen S, et al. Male and female genomes associated in a single pronucleus in human zygotes. *Biol Reprod.* 1995;52(3):653–657.
6. Papale L, Fiorentino A, Montag M, et al. Chapter 2: The zygote. Atlas of human embryology: from oocytes to preimplantation embryos. *Hum Reprod.* 2012;27(suppl 1):i22–i49.
7. Rosenbusch B, Schneider M, Glaseret B, et al. Cytogenetic analysis of giant oocytes and zygotes to assess their relevance for the development of digynic triploidy. *Hum Reprod.* 2002;17(9):2388–2392.
8. Rienzi L, Ubaldi F, Martinez F, et al. Relationship between meiotic spindle location with regard to the polar body position and oocyte developmental potential after ICSI. *Hum Reprod.* 2003;18(6):1289–1293.
9. Balakier H, Bouman D, Sojecki A, et al. Morphological and cytogenetic analysis of human giant oocytes and embryos. *Hum Reprod.* 2002;17(9):2394–2401.

9

Dynamic Aspects: Compaction

Sue Montgomery

Compaction is the process of increased cell-to-cell adhesion, followed by gap and tight junction formation between blastomeres, which in the human preimplantation embryo usually occurs after the third mitotic division. It is the first stage of differentiation in mammalian embryo development and can influence blastocyst formation and the differentiation of the first two cell lines: the inner cell mass cells that derive primarily the cells of the fetus, and the trophectoderm, the progenitor cells of the placenta.

The introduction of time-lapse technology into the IVF setting has revolutionized our ability to identify the exact time in hours post insemination (hpi), or in relation to another defined, key developmental time point. It is now feasible to identify the exact time that compaction is initiated, using the video footage to isolate the exact point, and time, that individual cell membranes first become indistinct (Figure 9.1). Video 9.1 shows embryo compaction and blastulation. The video can be viewed online: http://goo.gl/yd3eJW.

The use of time-lapse technology has demonstrated that the start time of compaction (hpi) can vary considerably, from as early as 50 to as late as 105 hpi (Figure 9.2). The duration of compaction may also vary. Whether or not this is related to viability needs to be established, but there is some evidence to suggest that delay in the onset of compaction results in reduced blastocyst development. Early compaction, in contrast, by day 3 of development, results in increased implantation rates.[1–3] Several recent time-lapse studies have found an association between compaction and ploidy of the resulting blastocyst.[4] A study of fragmented embryos at CARE Fertility identified that embryos that completed compaction in less than 22 hours were significantly more likely to result in euploid blastocysts.[5] Another recent abstract reported a similar phenomenon in all embryos, showing that the duration of compaction was around 5 hours longer in aneuploid embryos, compared with euploid.[6]

Time-lapse observation demonstrates that compaction is generally initiated in one part of the embryo and then quickly progresses across the whole embryo (Figure 9.1). It should be further noted here that the process of embryo fragmentation at the cleavage stage often impairs the compaction process, and this may affect development potential.

It is also apparent from time-lapse observation that the proportion of the embryo that participates in the compaction process can vary, and once concluded the compaction process can be defined as 'complete' (all cellular material incorporated) or 'incomplete' (some cellular material excluded). This phenomenon, of excluding material, is seen with cellular fragments as well as with intact cells (Figure 9.3). Preliminary data suggest that this may also be related to an embryo's ability to form a blastocyst and its implantation outcome, with embryos exhibiting complete compaction having a higher implantation potential.[1,7]

REFERENCES

1. Ivec M, Kovacic B, Vlaisavljevic V. Prediction of human blastocyst development from morulas with delayed and/or incomplete compaction. *Fertil Steril*. 2011;96:1473–1478.
2. Iwata K, Yumoto K, Sugishima M, et al. Analysis of compaction initiation in human embryos by using time-lapse cinematography, *J Assist Reprod Genet*. 2014;31(4):421–426.
3. Skiadas C, Jackson K, Racowsky C. Early compaction on day 3 may be associated with increased implantation potential. *Fertil Steril*. 2006;86:1386–1391.
4. Campbell A, Fishel S, Bowman N, et al. Modelling a risk classification of aneuploidy in human embryos using non-invasive morphokinetics. *Reprod BioMed Online*. 2013;26:477–485.
5. Montgomery S, Duffy S, Bowman N, et al. Does the duration of compaction differ in embryos that become euploid or aneuploid blastocysts? *Hum Reprod*. 2013 June;28:i1–i4.
6. Melzer K, Noyes N, Hodes-Wertz B, et al. How well do morphokinetic (MK) parameters and time-lapse microscopy (TLM) predict euploidy? A pilot study of TLM with trophectoderm (TE) biopsy with array comparative genomic hybridization. *Fertil Steril*. 2013;100(3, suppl):S209.
7. Power E, Montgomery S, Duffy S, et al. Can completion of compaction predict implantation outcome? *Hum Reprod*. 2013;28:i149–i206.

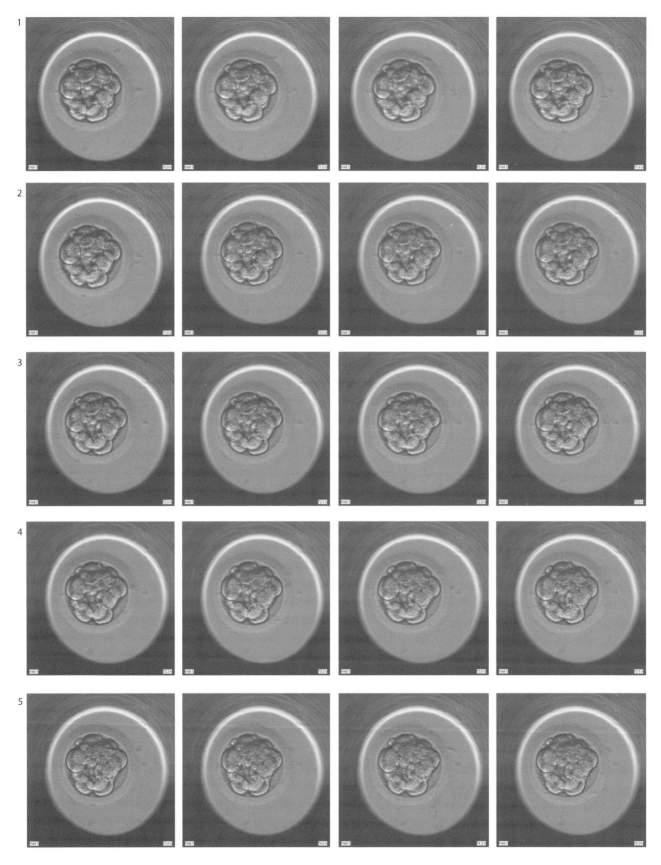

Figure 9.1 Initiation and progression of the compaction process. (Timings: row 1, panel 1, 70.9 h; row 2, panel 1, 71.5 h; row 3, panel 1, 72.5 h; row 4, panel 1, 73.2 h; row 5, panel 1, 73.8 h.)

(a)

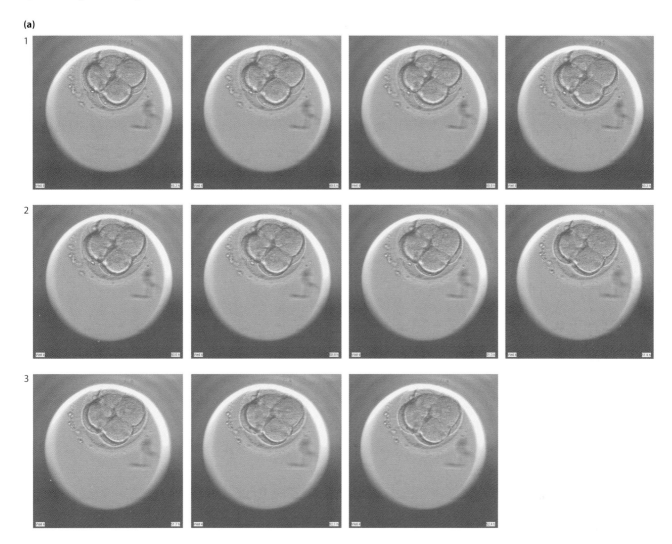

Figure 9.2a Initiation of compaction at 50 hpi. (Timings: row 1, panel 1, 49.3 h; row 2, panel 1, 50.6 h; row 3, panel 1, 51.7 h.)

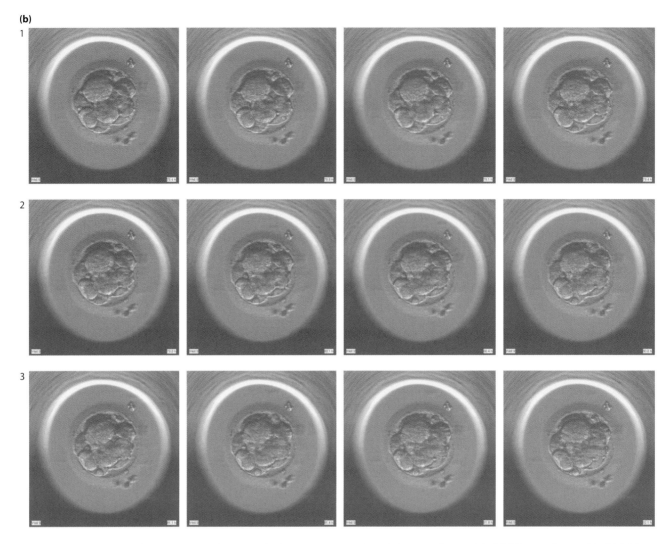

Figure 9.2b Initiation of compaction at 81 hpi. (Timings: row 1, panel 1, 78.4 h; row 2, panel 1, 79.8 h; row 3, panel 1, 81.1 h.)

(c)

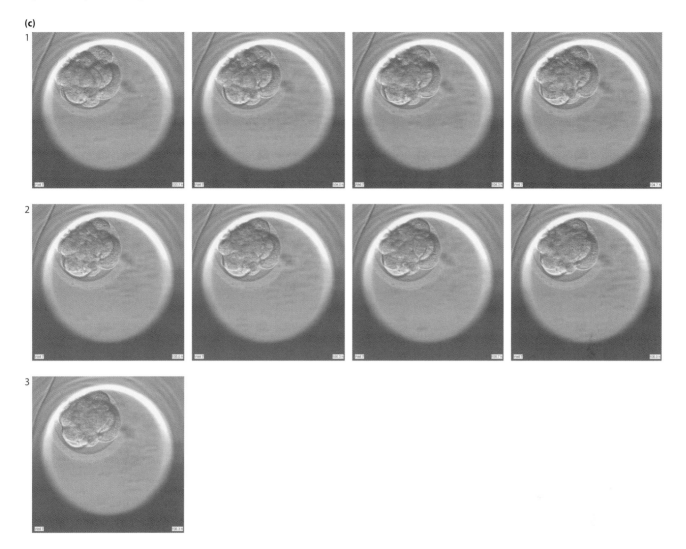

Figure 9.2c Initiation of compaction at 105 hpi. (Timings: row 1, panel 1, 103.7 h; row 2, panel 1, 105.0 h; row 3, panel 1, 103.6 h.)

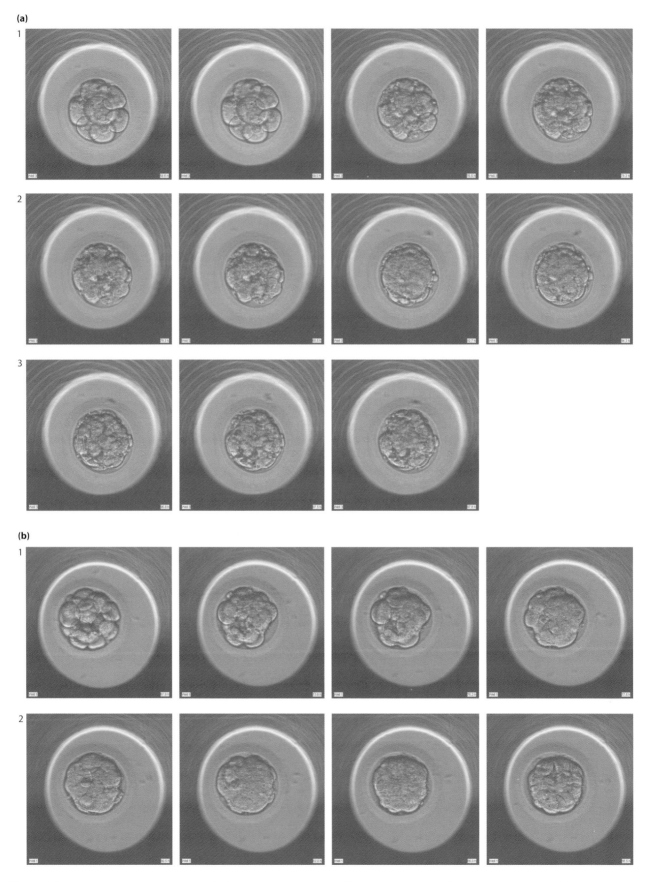

Figure 9.3 (a) Incomplete compaction. (Timings: row 1, panel 1, 58.6 h; row 2, panel 1, 79.3 h; row 3, panel 1, 96.8 h.) (b) Complete compaction. (Timings: row 1, panel 1, 67.9 h; row 2, panel 1, 80.5 h.)

10

Blastulation

Sue Montgomery

Blastulation is the process leading to the formation of a blastocoel, where the cells on the outside of the embryo polarize to form the trophectoderm (TE), creating an impermeable seal. Fluid is then transported to the extracellular spaces on the interior of the embryo, via sodium transport channels, causing blastocyst expansion. Tight junctions formed in the process of compaction prevent the leakage of fluid from the cavity. The inner cell mass (ICM) also becomes defined within the cavity.

Using time-lapse technology in the in vitro fertilization (IVF) setting, we can identify the exact time in hours post insemination (hpi) at which key events occur. In the case of blastulation it is feasible to identify the point that this process is initiated, if necessary by re-winding the video footage once a blastocyst has formed, identifying precisely the start time of cavity formation (Figure 10.1). Video 10.1 shows blastocyst expansion and collapse. The video can be viewed online: http://goo.gl/Rarlz4. Video 10.2 shows morphokinetic time points in embryo development. The video can be viewed online: http://goo.gl/ibWDjn.

From time-lapse observation it is demonstrated that the start time of blastulation can vary widely, from as early as 50 hpi to as late as 100 hpi (Figure 10.2). There is evidence to suggest that this may be related to implantation potential and the ploidy status of the embryo.[1] Those embryos that exhibit a delay in the start of blastulation may be less likely to implant and more likely to be aneuploid.

There is also a wide range in time that embryos reach the full blastocyst stage (tB), although this will be dependent on the definition given to this stage, which requires consistency. The definition for tB used by Campbell et al. was when the blastocoele filled the embryo with less than 10 percent increase in its diameter. In applying such a definition, we can observe a wide variation in the time after insemination that this stage is reached, from as early as 85 hpi to as late as 120 hpi (Figure 10.3). This has been shown to correlate to implantation potential and

ploidy status, with the late-forming blastocysts having a reduced implantation potential and a higher chance of aneuploidy compared with those reaching this stage earlier.[1,2]

Time-lapse imaging also facilitates quantitative assessment of the quality of the ICM and TE cells, which can vary widely. In most clinical programmes, blastocyst grading considers both cell lines and gives an independent grade to each.[3] For many years it was usually considered that the ICM grade was the most predictive of outcome, but recently there is growing evidence that the TE quality may be more predictive of implantation potential.[4,5]

Figure 10.4 shows the variation in quality of these two cell lines that can be observed.

REFERENCES

1. Campbell A, Fishel S, Bowman N, et al. Modelling a risk classification of aneuploidy in human embryos using non-invasive morphokinetics. *Reprod BioMed Online*. 2013;26: 477–485.
2. Campbell A, Fishel S, Bowman N, et al. Retrospective analysis of outcome after using an aneuploidy risk model derived from time-lapse imaging without PGS. *Reprod Biomed Online*. 2013;27:140–146.
3. Gardner D, Lane M, Stevens J, Schlenker T, Schoolcraft W. Blastocyst score affects implantation and pregnancy outcome: towards a single blastocyst transfer. *Fertil Steril*. 2000; 73(6):1155–1158.
4. Van der Wieden RM. Trophectoderm morphology grading reflects the interactions between embryo and endometrium. *Fertil Steril*. 2013;100(4):e1. doi: 10.1016/j.fertnstert.2012. 12.003. Epub 2013 Jan 8.
5. Hill MJ, Richter KS, Heitmann RJ, et al. Trophectoderm grade predicts outcomes of single blastocyst transfers. *Fertil Steril*. 2013 Apr;99(5):1283–1289.e1. Epub 2013 Jan 8.

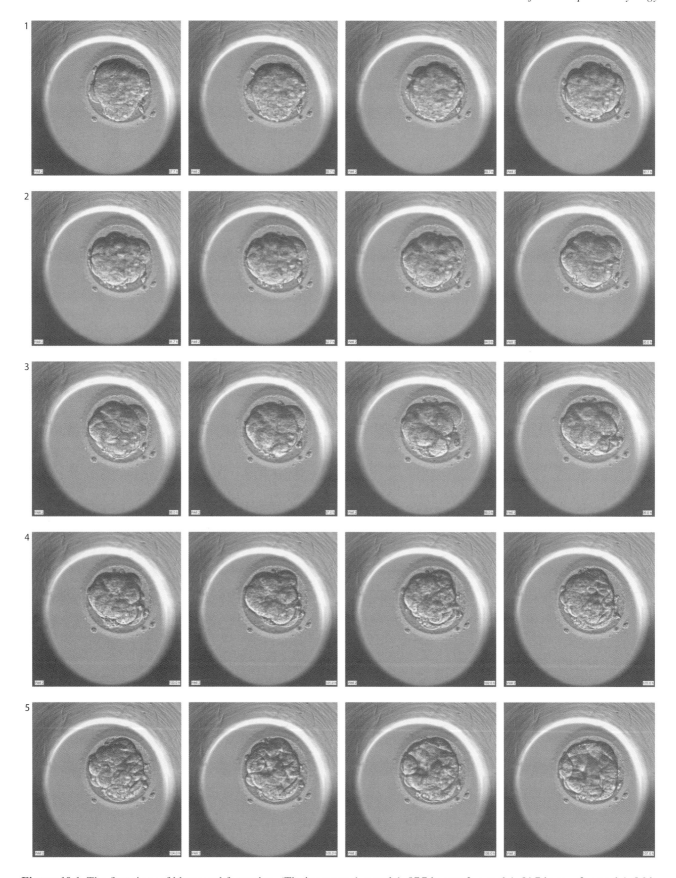

Figure 10.1 The first signs of blastocoel formation. (Timings: row 1, panel 1, 87.7 h; row 2, panel 1, 91.7 h; row 3, panel 1, 96 h; row 4, panel 1, 100 h; row 5, panel 1, 104 h.)

(a)

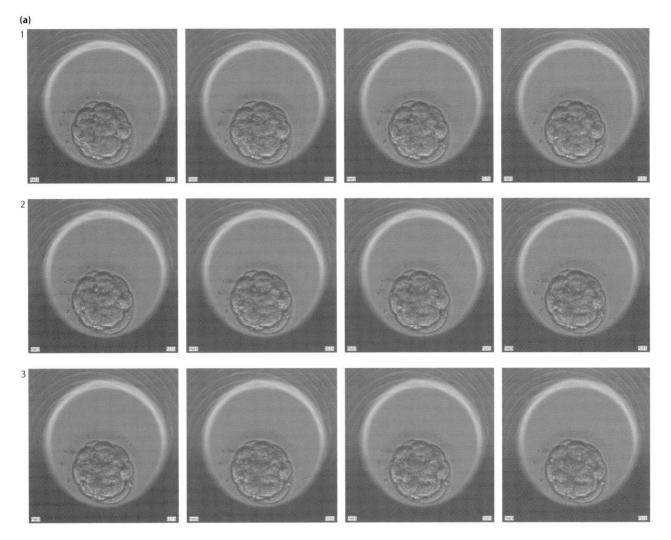

Figure 10.2a Varied start times of blastulation in hpi. (Timings: row 1, panel 1, 71.4 h; row 2, panel 1, 72 h; row 3, panel 1, 72.7 h.)

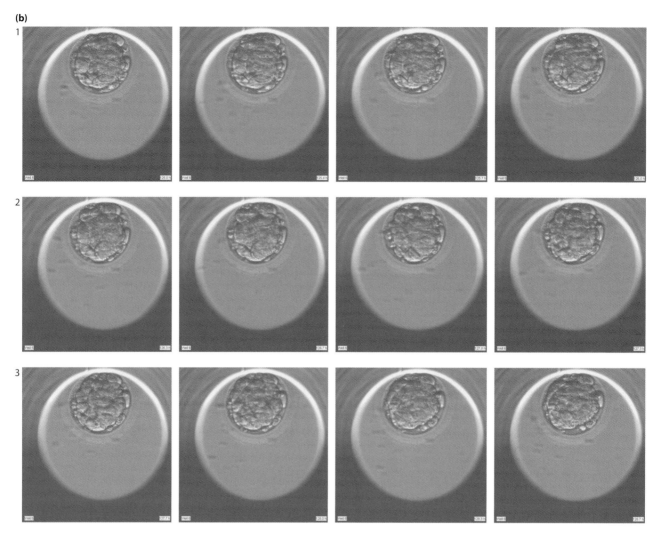

Figure 10.2b Varied start times of blastulation in hpi (continued). (Timings: row 1, panel 1, 125 h; row 2, panel 1, 126.3 h; row 3, panel 1, 127.7 h.)

(a)

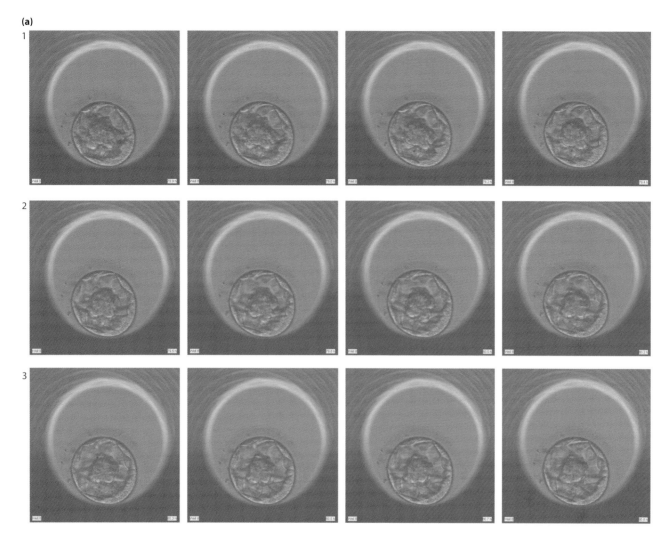

Figure 10.3a Variation in the time to reach full blast (atlas images). (Timings: row 1, panel 1, 78.9 h; row 2, panel 1, 79.5 h; row 3 panel 1, 80.3 h.)

(b)

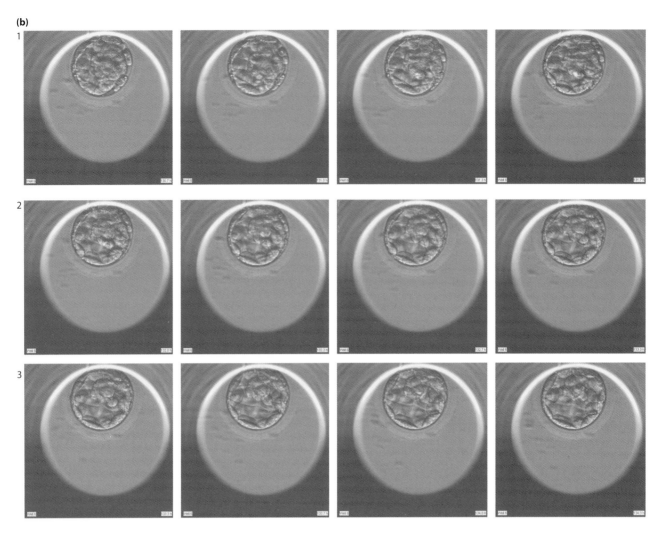

Figure 10.3b Variation in the time to reach full blast (continued). (Timings: row 1, panel 1, 130.7 h; row 2, panel 1, 132 h; row 3, panel 1, 133.3 h.)

(a)

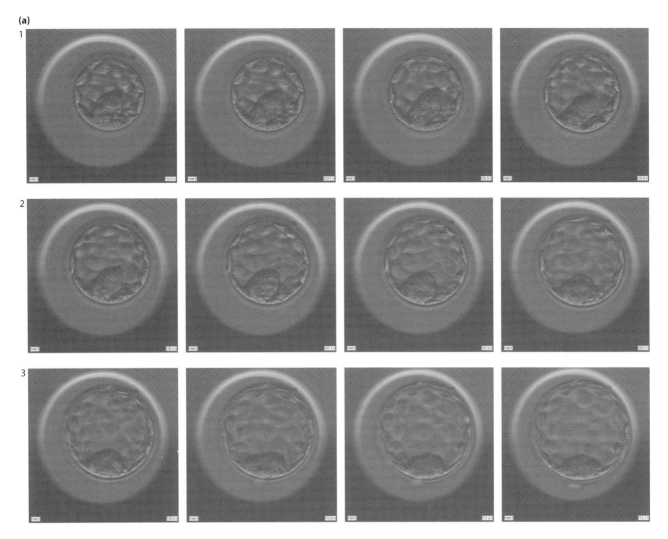

Figure 10.4a Varied morphologies of ICM and TE. (Timings: row 1, panel 1, 102.9 h; row 2, panel 1, 106.2 h; row 3, panel 1, 109.6 h.)

(b)

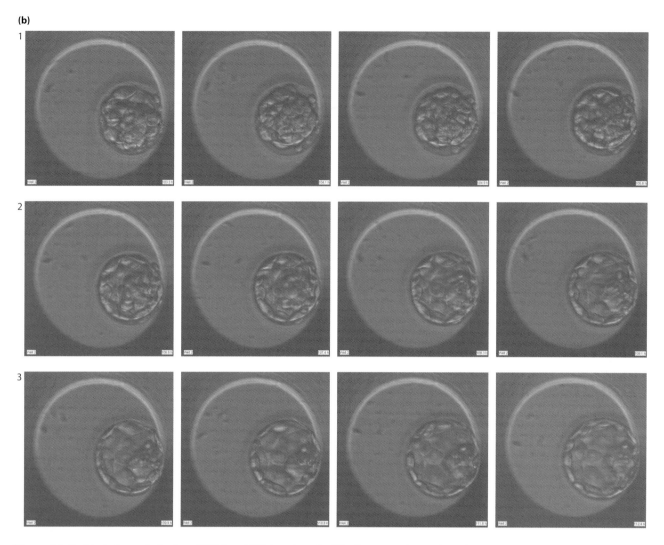

Figure 10.4b Varied morphologies of ICM and TE (continued). (Timings: row 1, panel 1, 103.3 h; row 2, panel 1, 106.6 h; row 3, panel 1, 109.9 h.)

(c)

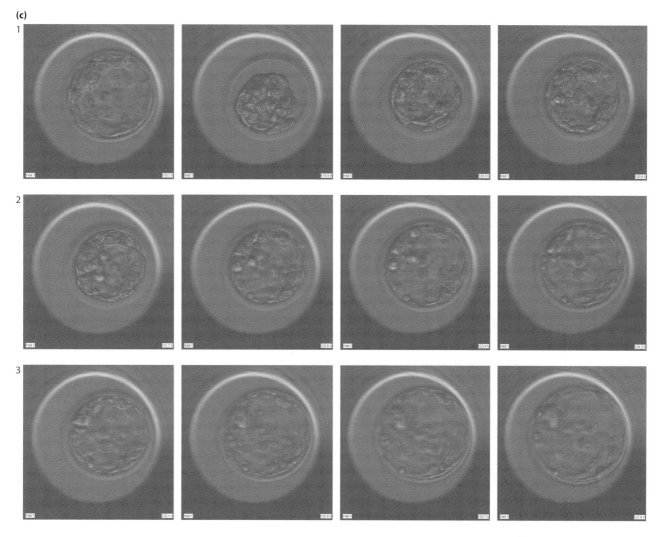

Figure 10.4c Varied morphologies of ICM and TE (continued). (Timings: row 1, panel 1, 118.1 h; row 2, panel 1, 121.7 h; row 3, panel 1, 125.1 h.)

11

Hatching of the Human Blastocyst

Louise Kellam

The human *zona pellucida* (ZP) is a gelatinous, extracellular matrix that surrounds oocytes and embryos until hatching and implantation. It is 15 to 20 μm thick and is formed in the early stages of ovarian follicular development by secretions from the oocyte and follicle granulosa cells.[1] It is a multilaminar structure composed primarily of four glycoproteins, designated ZP1, ZP2, ZP3, and ZP4, that are synthesized in primordial oocytes with each having specific roles in fertilization.[2] As well as regulating spermatozoa-egg interaction, the ZP has a critical role in gamete recognition and prevention of polyspermy. It also protects the embryo from immune cells and, acting as a physical retainer, prevents blastomeres dispersing during preimplantation development.[3] During formation of the blastocyst the embryo remains enclosed in the ZP. Prior to implantation, however, the expanded blastocyst must emerge out of the ZP to attach, adhere, and invade the receptive female uterine endometrium.[4] The emergence of the blastocyst from the ZP is referred to as *hatching*. Video 11.1 shows a blastocyst expanding and then hatching through the zona pellucida. The video can be viewed online: http://goo.gl/y0zYFA.

The in vivo hatching process is believed to differ from the in vitro equivalent as a result of interactions between the blastocyst and uterus. Little is known about the process in the human, but animal studies suggest in vivo hatching involves the presence of uterine zona lysins that assist the dissolution of the ZP and do not depend on blastocyst expansion.[5,6]

In vitro, however, an expanding blastocyst can hatch, unaided by uterine influences. The precise mechanisms are unknown, but it is a likely consequence of a combination of tension of periodic blastocyst contraction/expansion, actin-based modifications, and enzymatic digestion of trophectoderm cells.[7–9] This causes the blastocyst to gradually herniate out of the thinned ZP through an opening. The site of hatching is often observed at the pole opposite the inner cell mass, though a few hatch out at the embryo pole or elsewhere.[10] Different phenomena, such as trophectoderm projections, specialized cells named *zona breakers*, or localized effects of zona lysine proteases have all been suggested to assist hatching.[10–13] Once the blastocyst has fully emerged in vitro, the empty ZP can be observed with a single opening.

In Figure 11.1, the blastocyst is seen to collapse and a clear opening is apparent in the ZP at the 2-o'clock position. Although this appears similar to a mechanical breach, this was not due to any laboratory intervention, the blastocyst was undisturbed throughout in vitro culture. It seems the mechanical pressure of the swelling blastocoel cavity causes the

thinning ZP to rupture, creating an opening. This phenomenon appears to be directly associated with the subsequent collapse of the blastocyst as observed in other hatching blastocysts using time-lapse recordings (unpublished observations). The blastocyst re-expands, and by 124.7 hpi, it begins to herniate through the established ZP opening created approximately 2 hours earlier, at the opposite pole to the inner cell mass (Figure 11.1b). At 125.6 hpi, a number of trophectoderm cells emerge through the ZP while the blastocyst remains fully expanded (Figure 11.1c). Despite this initial protrusion of cells, the blastocyst collapses again, and cellular material can be seen between the ZP opening and the retracting trophectoderm. By 126.6 hpi, following another re-expansion phase, the trophectoderm herniates through the ZP for a second time (Figure 11.1d). No subsequent collapse is observed.

Subsequently (Figure 11.2), an increasing amount of trophectoderm pushes through the ZP breach while the blastocyst remains in an expanded state. At approximately 133.6 hpi, the volume of the herniating trophoblast appears similar in volume to the remaining blastocyst within the ZP (Figure 11.2a). Expansion of the ZP is reduced, perhaps as a consequence of a shift in pressure into the zona-free protruding trophoblast cells. By 136.6 hpi the increasing overall size of the hatching blastocyst has caused it to change position within the microwell. The trophectoderm begins to come away from the inner walls, and the inner cell mass remains within (Figure 11.2b). By 140.6 hpi only the inner cell mass appears to remain in the zona pellucida; the rest of the herniated trophectoderm has expanded to a size outside the camera field of view (Figure 11.2c). This hatching blastocyst was vitrified at this stage.

In approximately 25 to 30 percent of human embryos cultured in vitro, hatching generally occurs between day 5 and 6 post oocyte recovery and is a favourable prognostic factor for in vitro fertilization (IVF) outcome.[14–16] Dysregulation of the hatching process causes implantation failure leading to infertility.[17] Methods to assist hatching and encourage implantation have been employed clinically, including partial mechanical zona dissection, zona drilling, zona thinning, and mechanical expansion, making use of acid tyrodes, proteinases, piezon vibrator manipulators, and lasers. The aim of these techniques is to overcome what has been termed *zona hardening*, a consequence of IVF or cryopreservation (described further in Chapter 18, Zona Defects). Other reasons given for assisted hatching are to enhance hormonal and metabolite exchange and messaging between the embryo and the endometrium.[18] The clinical effectiveness of assisted hatching prior to embryo transfer is

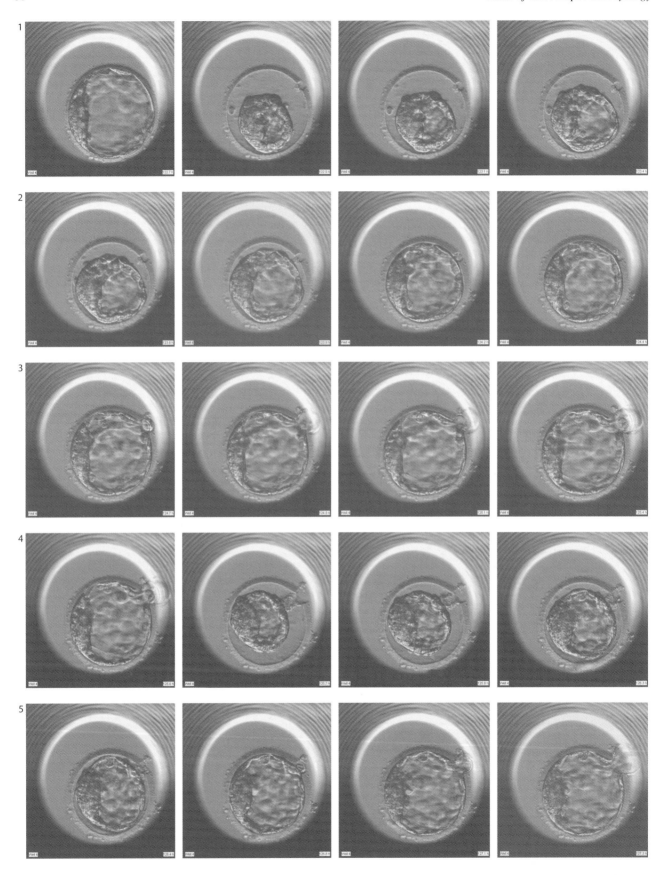

Figure 11.1 Series of time-lapse images at 10-minute intervals. (Timings: row 1, panel 1, 122.7 hpi; row 2, panel 1, 123.6 h; row 3, panel 1, 124.7 h; row 4, panel 1, 125.6 h; row 5, panel 1, 126.4 h.)

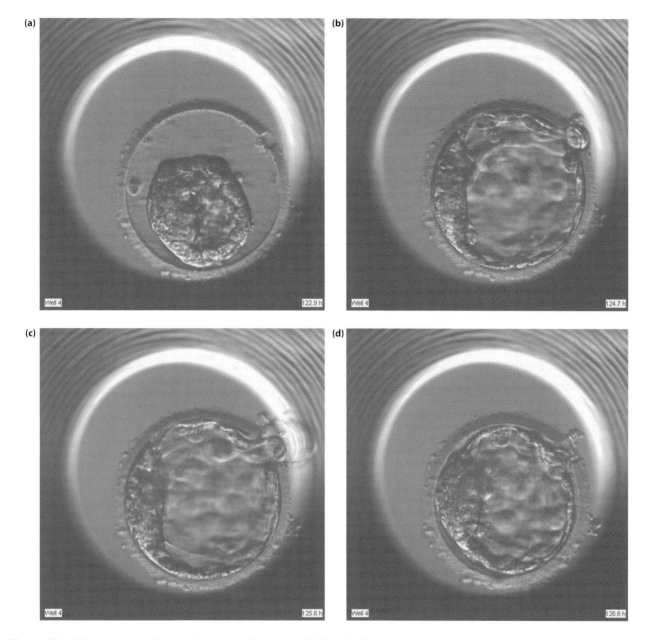

Figure 11.1 (Continued.) (a) Enlarged version of image at 122.9 h. (b) Enlarged version of image at 124.7 h. (c) Enlarged version of image at 125.6 h. (d) Enlarged version of image at 126.6 h.

contentious. A Cochrane review of 31 assisted hatching studies found there was no significant difference in the odds of live birth in the assisted hatching group compared with the control group, and it is argued as to whether there is any clinical benefit.[19] Assisted hatching has the possible hazard of depriving the embryo of immune protection from the ZP; however, an improvement in clinical implantation by a once commonly used treatment involving immune suppressants is debatable.[20,21] Many clinics, including CARE Fertility, no longer perform assisted hatching except in the rare case of an abnormally thick zona. (See images in Chapter 18, Zona Defects.)

Rarely, two or more sites of hatching have been observed in vitro.[22] It has been suggested that this might arise in intracytoplasmic sperm injection (ICSI)-generated blastocysts due to incomplete closure of the zona breach created by the microinjection pipette.[23] Even with time-lapse monitoring of oocytes post ICSI, tracking the site of the breach on the ZP to confirm this phenomena would, at present, be a challenge. Hatching at more than one point in the ZP, particularly when one of the holes is very small, could result in trapping of the blastocyst within the ZP as the pressure within the blastocoel cavity would be dissipated and not concentrated on one hatching site. Manipulation of the ZP has been associated with an increased risk of monozygotic twinning possibly due to the physical restriction on the emerging embryo causing it to split.[24]

The complete absence of a ZP has been reported in some oocytes of infertile women, reflecting its importance. However, a case report of a zona-free (corona cell intact) pregnancy following ICSI suggests that the coronal cells may provide sufficient support to maintain blastomere interaction and embryo

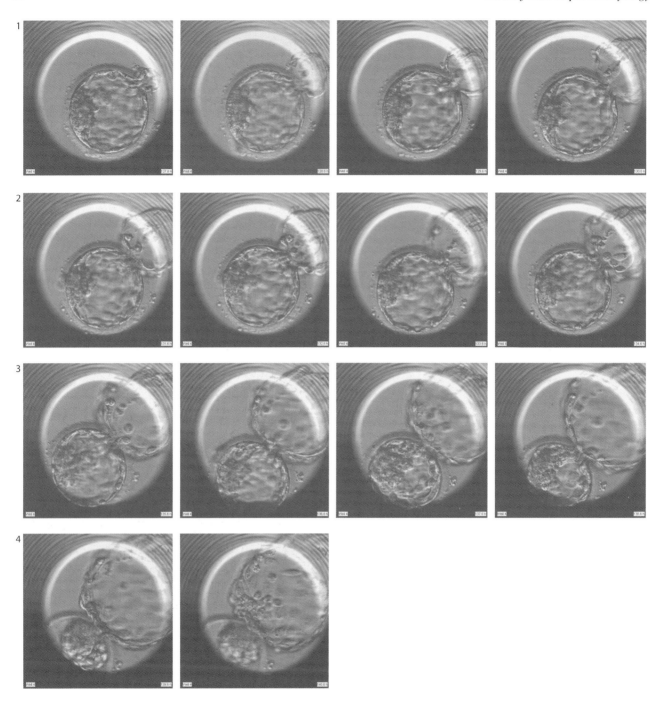

Figure 11.2 The same blastocyst as in Figure 11.1 with blastocyst hatching from 126.6 hpi, yet at 1-hour intervals. (Timings: row 1, panel 1, 127.6 h; row 2, panel 1, 131.6 h; row 3, panel 1, 135.6 h; row 4, panel 1, 139.6 h.)

viability, with the ZP not necessarily essential for early embryo development and pregnancy.[25]

Hatched human blastocysts have been transferred to the uterus successfully, and there is evidence to suggest that transfer of spontaneously hatching or hatched blastocyst yields better pregnancy rates than nonhatching expanded blastocyst transfer.[16,23] In practice, where standard policy is to transfer blastocysts on day 5 or day 6, the likelihood of observing spontaneously fully hatching blastocysts is very low. The incidence may be higher in previously vitrified/warmed blastocysts, or those that

have undergone blastomere or trophectoderm biopsy, where the ZP will have been compromised (Figure 11.3).

Differences in the hatching mechanisms between blastomere-biopsied embryos and nonbiopsied embryos have been observed in time-lapse studies. Blastocysts in the biopsied group escaped through the artificially induced hole in a thick ZP instead of being preceded by the gradual thinning of the ZP in the expanding blastocysts in the control group.[26] Some authors, using mouse and cattle embryos, believe early extrusion of the blastocyst through the induced ZP breach has a negative effect on the embryo,

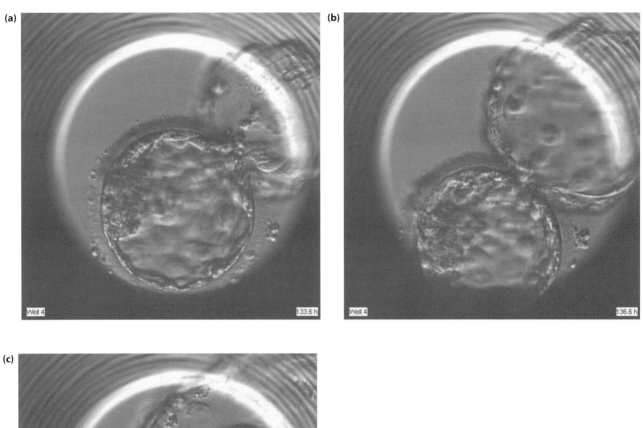

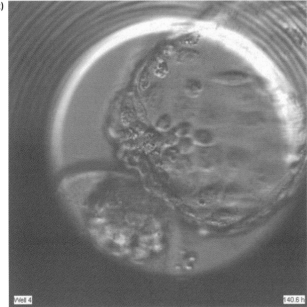

Figure 11.2 (Continued.) (a) Enlarged version of image at 133.6 h. (b) Enlarged version of image at 136.6 h. (c) Enlarged version of image at 140.6 h.

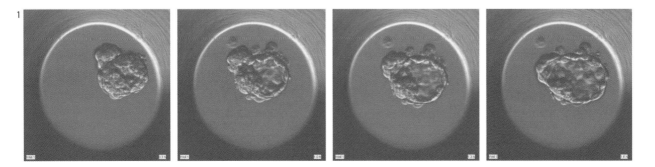

Figure 11.3 Time-lapse images showing the expansion of a fully hatched blastocyst post embryo biopsy, vitrification, and then warming. This embryo was subsequently transferred, resulting in a normal live birth. (Timings: row 1, panel 1, 0.3 h.)

although this depends on the size and number of holes introduced.[27–29] In a clinical setting, the alternative embryo biopsy approach of removing trophectoderm cells through a breach in the zona at the blastocyst stage avoids an earlier facilitative zona breach at the cleavage stage which may benefit the embryo.[30]

Further time-lapse studies looking at the site, timing, and mechanism of human blastocyst hatching, with and without intervention, will contribute to our understanding of this extraordinary process, both in vitro and in vivo.

REFERENCES

1. Rankin T, Dean J. The molecular genetics of the zona pellucida: mouse mutations and infertility. *Hum Reprod.* 1996;2:889–894.
2. Lefièvre L, Conner SJ, Salpekar A, et al. Four zona pellucida glycoproteins are expressed in the human. *Hum Reprod.* 2004;19:1580–1586.
3. Wassarman PM, Jovine L, Qi H, et al. Recent aspects of mammalian fertilization research. *Mol Cell Endocrinol.* 2005;234:95–103.
4. Seshagiri PB, Roy SS, Sireesha G, et al. Cellular and molecular regulation of mammalian blastocyst hatching. *J Reprod Immunol.* 2009;83:79–84.
5. Gonzales D, Bavister BD. *Zona pellucida* escape by hamster blastocysts in vitro is delayed and morphologically different compared with zona escape in vivo. *Biol Reprod.* 1995;52:470–480.
6. Rosenfeld MG, Joshi MD. Effect of a rat uterine fluid endopeptidase on lysis of the zona pellucida. *J Reprod Fertil.* 1981;61:199–203.
7. Montag M, Koll B, Holmes P, et al. Significance of the number of embryonic cells and the state of the zona pellucida for hatching of mouse blastocysts in vitro versus in vivo. *Biol Reprod.* 2000;62:1738–1744.
8. Schiewe MC, Hazeleger NL, Sclimenti C, et al. Physiological characterization of blastocyst hatching mechanisms by use of a mouse antihatching model. *Fertil Steril.* 1995b;63:288–294.
9. Bazer FW, Spencer TE, Johnson GA, et al. Comparative aspects of implantation. *Reproduction.* 2009;138:195–209.
10. Sathananthan H, Menezes J, Gunasheela S. Mechanics of human blastocyst hatching in vitro. *Reprod Biomed Online.* 2003 Sep;7(2):228–234.
11. Gonzales DS, Jones JM, Pinyopummintr T, et al. Trophectoderm projections: a potential means for locomotion, attachment and implantation of bovine, equine and human blastocysts. *Hum Reprod.* 1996;11:2739–2745.
12. O'Sullivan CM, Rancourt SL, Liu SY, et al. A novel murine tryptase involved in blastocyst hatching and outgrowth. *Reproduction.* 2001;122:61–71.
13. Sharma N, Liu S, Tang L, Irwin J, Meng G, Rancourt DE. Implantation serine proteinases heterodimerize and are critical in hatching and implantation. *BMC Dev Biol.* 2006;6:61.
14. Gardner DK, Lane M, Kouridakis K, et al. Complex physiological base serum-free culture media increase mammalian embryo development. In: Gomel V, Leung PCK (eds). *In vitro fertilization and assisted reproduction.* Bologna: Monduzzi Editore; 1997:551–554.
15. Yoon HJ, Yoon SH, Son WY, et al. High implantation and pregnancy rates with transfer of human hatching day 6 blastocysts. *Fertil Steril.* 2001 Apr;75(4):832–833.
16. Chimote NM, Chimote NN, Nath NM, Mehta BN. Transfer of spontaneously hatching or hatched blastocyst yields better pregnancy rates than expanded blastocyst transfer. *J Hum Reprod Sci.* 2013 Jul–Sep;6(3):183–188.
17. Petersen CG, Mauri AL, Baruffi RL, et al. Implantation failures: success of assisted hatching with quarter-laser zona thinning. *Reprod Biomed Online.* 2005;10:224–229.
18. Cohen J, Alikani M, Trowbridge J, et al. Implantation enhancement by selective assisted hatching using zona drilling of human embryos with poor prognosis. *Hum Reprod.* 1992;7(5):685–691.
19. Carney S-K, Das S, Blake D, et al. Assisted hatching on assisted conception (in vitro fertilisation (IVF) and intracytoplasmic sperm injection (ICSI)). *Cochrane Database Syst Rev.* 2012;12:Cd001894. doi: 10.1002/14651858.Cd001894.Pub5
20. Cohen J, Malter H, Elsner C, et al. Immunosuppression supports implantation of zona pellucida dissected human embryos. *Fertil Steril.* 1990 Apr;53(4):662–665.
21. Lee KA, Koo JJ, Yoon TK, et al. Immunosuppression by corticosteroid has no effect on the pregnancy rate in routine in-vitro fertilization/embryo transfer patients. *Hum Reprod.* 1994 Oct;9(10):1832–1835.
22. Fong CY, Bongso A, Sathananthan H, et al. Ultrastructural observations of enzymatically treated human blastocysts: zona-free blastocyst transfer and rescue of blastocysts with hatching difficulties. *Hum Reprod.* 2001;16:540–546.
23. Fong C, Bongso A, Ng S, et al. Ongoing normal pregnancy after transfer of zona-free blastocysts: implications for embryo transfer in the human. *Hum Reprod.* 1997;12(3):557–560.
24. Cohen J, Elsner C, Kort H, et al. Impairment of the hatching process following IVF in the human and improvement of implantation by assisting hatching using micromanipulation. *Hum Reprod.* 1990 Jan;5(1):7–13.
25. Stanger J, Stevenson K, Lakmaker A, et al. Pregnancy following fertilization of zona-free, coronal cell intact human ova: case report. *Hum Reprod.* 2001;16(1):164–167.
26. Kirkegaard K, Hindkjaer J, Ingerslev J. Human embryonic development after blastomere removal: a time-lapse analysis. *Hum Reprod.* 2012;27(1):97–105.
27. Schmoll F, Schneider H, Montag M, et al. Effects of different laser-drilled openings in the zona pellucida on hatching of in vitro-produced cattle blastocysts. *Fertil Steril.* 2003;80 (suppl):714–719.
28. Duncan FE, Stein P, Williams CJ, et al. The effect of blastomere biopsy on preimplantation mouse embryo development and global gene expression. *Fertil Steril.* 2009;91:1462–1465.
29. Cohen J, Feldberg D. Effects of the size and number of zona pellucida openings on hatching and trophoblast outgrowth in the mouse embryo. *Mol Reprod Dev.* 1991;30:70–78.
30. Scott R, Upham K, Forman E, et al. Cleavage-stage biopsy significantly impairs human embryonic implantation potential while blastocyst biopsy does not: a randomized and paired clinical trial. *Fertil Steril.* 2013 Sept;100(3): 624–630.

12

Irregular Cleavages

Kathryn Berrisford and Ellen Cater

Irregular cleavage events can be identified in the preimplantation human embryo using time-lapse imaging.

They are difficult to detect with standard discrete or *static* observation due to their dynamic nature and the transience of nuclear appearance and fading. With time-lapse imaging, it is possible to distinguish between three blastomeres, and two blastomeres with a large anucleate fragment, by observing the embryo during the phase of the cycle when the nuclei are visible and by the dynamics of the cleavage event. Video 12.1 shows an embryo demonstrating multinucleation and irregular cleavage. The video can be viewed online: http://goo.gl/D3X0Xl.

The duration of a normal cell cycle has not been accurately defined but requires sufficient time for DNA replication and cytokinesis. Extremely short cell cycles, therefore, could result in incomplete DNA replication, which may be associated with an unequal distribution of DNA to blastomeres.

Irregular cleavage may be defined by timing (very short or very long) or by pattern and may be distinguished using time lapse which is important as they are likely to be associated with differing biological events.

Irregular cleavage may be caused by a number of mechanisms including failure of extrusion of the second polar body, diploid gametes, or abnormalities in spindle formation. The centrioles that control the first mitotic divisions of the oocyte are introduced by the spermatozoan. Defective male centrosomes inherited by the zygote may lead to abnormal cleavage and compromised embryonic development.[4] Therefore, quality of the sperm (midpiece) can influence the formation of abnormal spindles during early cleavage of embryos. Also, any damage to the midpiece during intracytoplasmic sperm injection (ICSI) can be the cause of abnormal early embryo cleavage.[4]

Direct Cleavage

Direct cleavage (multichotomous mitosis) describes an irregular cleavage whereby one blastomere divides directly into three or more daughter blastomeres. However, the term *direct cleavage* was first used in 2012 following time-lapse studies of human preimplantation embryos to describe a fast division from two to three blastomeres in under 5 hours and was reported to occur at any cleavage stage.[1] This could, arguably, be more accurately named 'rapid cleavage'. Direct cleavage from one to three cells is most easily seen during the first and second mitotic cleavage cycles (i.e., zygote to three cells, or two cells to five or six cells)

and can occur with or without multinucleation. It may be associated with errors in spindle apparatus, for example, tripolar. It can be identified by calculations from time lapse records of cleavage events, for example if t3-t2 = 0, when the embryo did not, at least observably within the acquired images, exist at the two-cell stage as it cleaved directly to three cells.

Zaninovic and colleagues reported direct cleavage in 12 percent of embryos: 58 percent at first cleavage, 25 percent at second cleavage, and 6.7 percent at third cleavage division.[2] This group reported that overall development was impaired when direct cleavage had occurred and that only 9 percent of such embryos reached the blastocyst stage and were cryopreserved. Direct cleavage at the first cleavage resulted in poorer embryo development than later-stage onsets (second or third cleavages). Chromosome abnormalities were detected in 89 percent of direct-cleavage embryos, including different patterns of chromosomal aberrations unspecific for maternal or paternal origin. This large study noted an absence of triploidy within the direct-cleaving cohort, but division patterns of 3PN zygotes have previously been studied by Kola.[3] Most of these cleaved directly to three cells at the first cleavage and resulted in abnormal chromosomal content.

In Figure 12.1, the second polar body was extruded, and two pronuclei appeared and faded. The zygote then directly cleaved into three cells. In this example, following preimplantation genetic screening (PGS) analysis of a blastomere, the embryo was found to be affected by multiple aneuploidies.

Rapid Cleavage

Rapid cleavage (defined by Rubio et al.[1] as direct cleavage, from two to three blastomeres, in less than 5 hours) was demonstrated to be one of the most conclusive embryo de-selection parameters, reported to occur in approximately 14 percent of all embryos studied. Evidence suggests that such embryos have low implantation potential; therefore, their selection for transfer should be avoided, where possible.[1]

As the duration of a normal cell cycle has yet to be defined, rapid cleavage cannot be annotated, unless an arbitory value is introduced, as in the work by Rubio et al.[1] which used 5 hours. Rather, the durations associated with cleavages can be calculated from the annotation of the embryo reaching sequential cell stages, and when the normal cell cycle duration is defined, rapid cleavage can be identified against normal limits and based on clinical evidence.

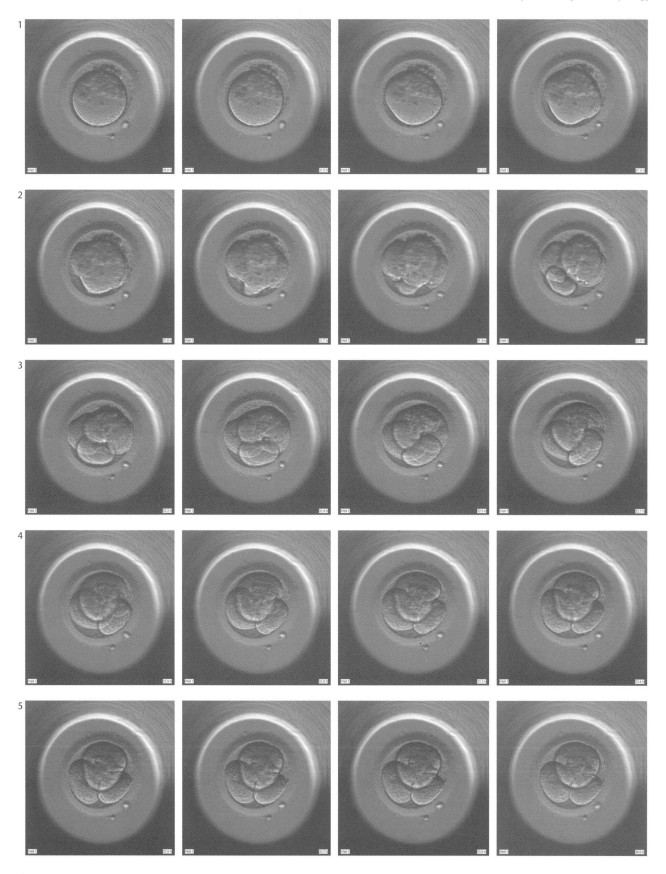

Figure 12.1 Direct division one to three cells. (Timings: row 1, panel 1, 30.9 h; row 1, panel 1, 31.5 h; row 3, panel 1, 32.2 h; row 4, panel 1, 32.9 h; row 5, panel 1, 33.5 h.)

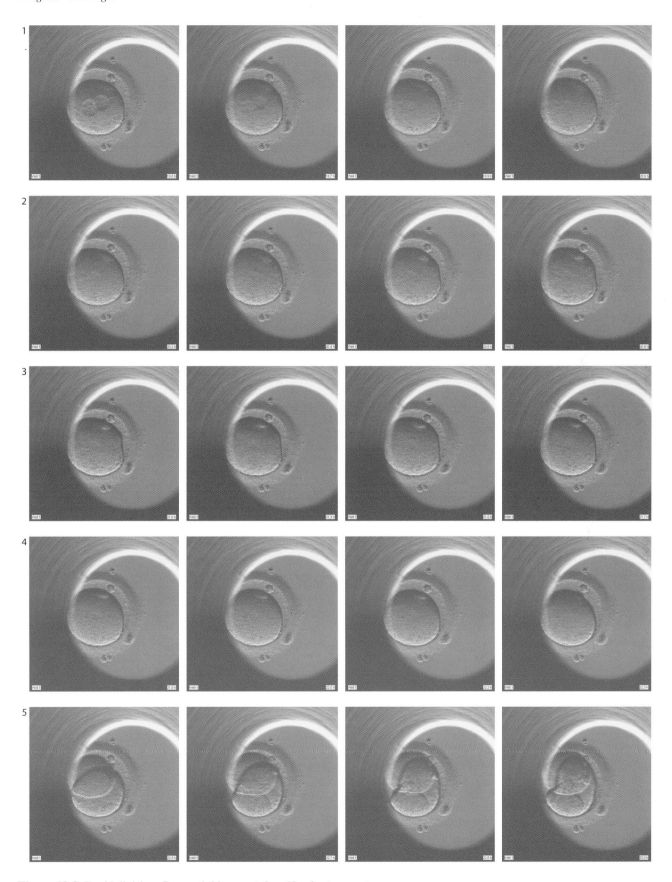

Figure 12.2 Rapid division. Sequential images taken 10 minutes apart.

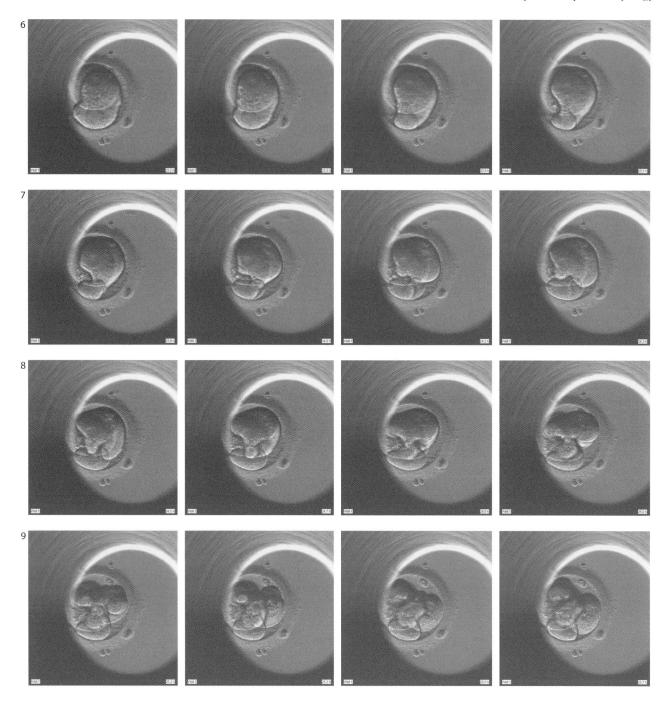

Figure 12.2 (Continued)

To fully understand the phenomenon of irregular cleavage, more analysis is necessary. To date, there are no studies that consider the incidence of this phenomenon in different patient groups or according to insemination or culture methods.

In Figure 12.2, the embryo progresses through the second cell cycle in less than 5 hours.

REFERENCES

1. Rubio I, Kuhlmann R, Agerholm I, et al. Limited implantation success of direct-cleaved human zygotes: a time-lapse study. *Fertil Steril.* 2012;98:1458–1463.

2. Zaninovic N, Ye Z, Zhan Q, et al. Cell stage onsets, embryo developmental potential and chromosomal abnormalities in embryos exhibiting direct unequal cleavages (DUCs). *Fertil Steril.* 2013;100(3) P S242. ASRM, Boston.

3. Kola I, Trounson A, Dawson G, et al. Tripronuclear human oocytes: altered cleavage patterns and subsequent karyotypic analysis of embryos. *Biol Reprod.* 1987;37:395-401.

4. Sathananthan J. Paternal centrosomal dynamics in early human development and infertility. *Assist Reprod Genet.* 1998;15:129–139.

13

Reverse Cleavage/Blastomere Fusion

Davina Hulme

Time-lapse observations of embryo development have shown that some cleavage-stage embryos reduce in cell number, a process referred to as *reverse cleavage* or *blastomere fusion*. In the majority of cases, two blastomeres of an embryo fuse resulting in a hybrid cell containing two nuclei (Figure 13.1). Video 13.1 shows irregular cell division and blastomere fusion. The video can be viewed online: http://goo.gl/rJMc5p.

Reverse cleavage is not well documented in the literature; however, Hickman and colleagues observed reverse cleavage in 6.8 percent of embryos, occurring between 24 and 136 hpi (hours post insemination), using time-lapse observations.[1] Of the embryos that reached the blastocyst stage, reverse cleavage occurred between 24 and 89 hpi. The study also indicated a link between reverse cleavage and multinucleation as there was a greater incidence of multinucleation ($p < 0.01$) in embryos that had undergone reverse cleavage compared with embryos with mononucleated cells. These authors also postulated that the mechanism controlling reverse cleavage may be susceptible to the environment of the oocyte during folliculogenesis; the embryos from GnRH antagonist cycles showed a lower reverse cleavage rate (2.8 percent) compared to the proportion of embryos derived from a long agonist downregulation (5.7 percent). Reverse cleavage did not seem to impair embryo development to the blastocyst stage and was not linked to ploidy status. Fragmentation, cell evenness, and morphokinetics were not affected by whether the embryo reverse cleaved or not.

Balakier et al. looked at the incidence of blastomere fusion after cryopreservation and thawing of early cleavage embryos, from static images.[2] They reported that depending upon the number of fused cells per embryo, blastomere fusion transformed the embryos into either entirely polyploid embryos (complete fusion at two- or three-cell stage) or into mosaics, being a mixture of polyploid and normal cells. They observed blastomere fusion at all developmental stages (2 to 10 cells), and the frequency was 4.6 percent in day 2 and 1.5 percent in day 3 thawed embryos. The study also suggests that blastomere fusion can affect morphologically good embryos (70 percent of embryos affected by blastomere fusion were *good quality* embryos). It is possible that a defect in the cell membrane is a prerequisite for initiation of such blastomere fusion, which can be induced by many membrane-disrupting agents such as a virus or specifically, as in the Balakier et al. study, by those used in freezing and thawing. It was postulated that abnormal cells resulting from fusion may be sequestered to the trophoblast and later the placenta.[2]

Further research is needed to determine the clinical significance of reverse-cleaved embryos and the molecular mechanisms that cause embryos to reverse cleave. At CARE Fertility, to date, 3.2 percent (445/13 823) of cleaved embryos exhibited blastomere fusion. Only 1.6 percent (62/3761) of embryos chosen for transfer had reverse cleaved. Of those with known implantation data (KID) 28.3 per cent (17/60) implanted (KID+) compared with a KID+ rate of 38.3 percent where no blastomere fusion was recorded. Live birth data following blastomere fusion is being collected and to date we report 17 live births (unpublished data). Stecher et al. have also reported a live birth from a day 5 embryo showing 'divisions back and forward to a 2-cell.'[3] This indicates that although they may have a reduced implantation potential, it is still possible to achieve a healthy live birth; however, it remains a recommended exclusion criterion when choosing embryos for transfer until further data are collected.

REFERENCES

1. Hickman CFL, Campbell A, Duffy S, et al. Reverse cleavage: its significance with regards to human embryo morphokinetics, ploidy and stimulation protocol. *Hum Reprod.* 2012; 27(suppl 2):ii103–ii105.
2. Balakier H, Cabaca O, Bouman D, et al. Spontaneous blastomere fusion after freezing and thawing of early human embryos leads to polyploidy and chromosomal mosaicism. *Hum Reprod.* 2000;15(11):2404–2410.
3. Stecher A, Vanderzwalmen P, Zintz M, et al. Transfer of blastocysts with deviant morphological and morphokinetic parameters at early stages of in-vitro development: a case series. *Reprod Biomed Online.* 2014;28(4):424–435.

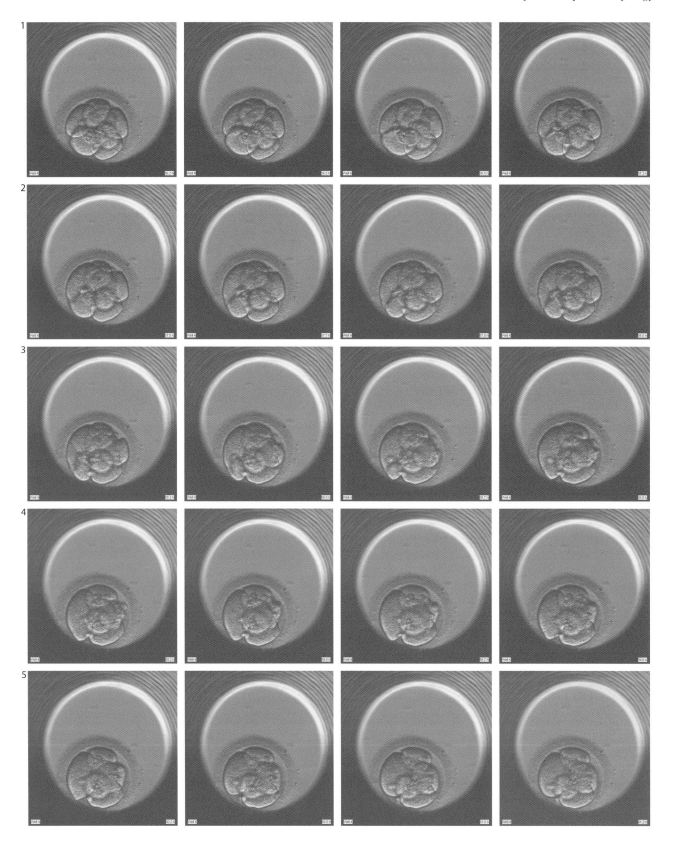

Figure 13.1 Series of time-lapse images, mostly at 10-minute intervals, showing two blastomeres of an eight-cell embryo fuse or reverse cleave. (Timings: row 1, panel 1, 56.2 h; row 2, panel 1, 57.5 h; row 3, panel 1, 58.2 h; row 4, panel 1, 59.2 h; row 5, panel 1, 60.2 h.)

14

Smooth Endoplasmic Reticulum Clusters

Cath Drezet

After the removal of the cumulus cells from the oocyte complexes prior to intracytoplasmic sperm injection (ICSI), translucent vacuoles of similar size to pronuclei are sometimes seen in metaphase II oocytes. These vacuoles are membrane-free accumulations, or aggregations, of smooth endoplasmic reticulum (sERC). sERCs differ from nuclei, pronuclei, and vacuoles as they exhibit a particularly glassy, or smooth, appearance, and they are void of nucleoli or visible matter within them (Figure 14.1). Video 14.1 shows a large sERC in the oocyte cytoplasm. The video can be viewed online: http://goo.gl/8ujnQM.

The presence of sERC is believed to indicate cytoplasmic damage and has been shown to be associated with decreased implantation rates and high miscarriage rates.[1,2] The ALPHA and ESHRE Istanbul Consensus 2011 recommend that oocytes with sERC should not be inseminated as there is risk of a significantly abnormal outcome including, for example, certain imprinting disorders (e.g., Beckwith-Wiedemann syndrome[1]). Cohorts of oocytes where some contain sERC can have overall normal fertilization rates and can produce morphologically normal embryos, but the clinical pregnancy rate is reduced, even if only sERC-negative embryos are replaced.

Figures 14.2 to 14.7 show a pronuclear-sized sERC moving around the egg, post injection. This egg showed no signs of fertilization. The sERC development is thought to be a result of high estradiol levels during stimulation and abnormal regulation of Ca 2+ signaling.[1] It has been proposed that it may be possible to avoid sERCs in subsequent cycles by using an alternative stimulation method or by giving the final hCG injection earlier in the treatment cycle where sERC was previously observed. Miwa et al. showed the presence of sERC in at least one oocyte in 7.3 percent of stimulated cycles, of which 89.1 percent went on to have sERC-negative cycles with a subsequent modification of stimulation regime.[3] Ebner et al. reported that 1.8 percent of oocytes were affected by sERC and found a direct correlation between stimulation dose and duration, leading to significantly reduced fertilization and blastulation rates.[4]

The presence of sERC is one of the few oocyte dysmorphisms to result in a negative influence on the postimplantation development of the embryo. However, a recent study reported that sERC-positive embryos have the capacity to develop into normal pregnancies, resulting in seven healthy babies.[5] More research into sERC is required to clarify whether or not these

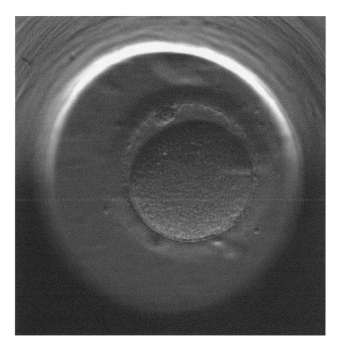

Figure 14.1 sERC at 15.9 h post injection.

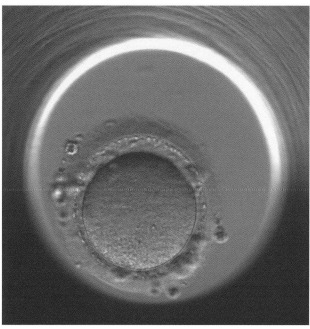

Figure 14.2 The sERC 28.8 h post injection.

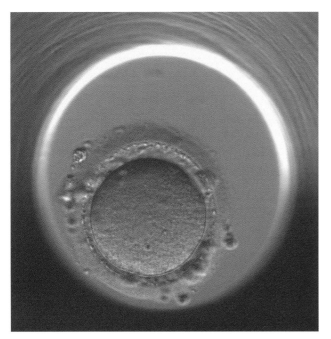

Figure 14.3 The sERC 29.1 h post injection.

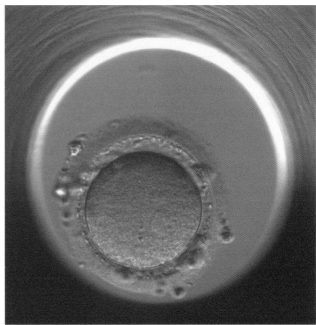

Figure 14.5 The sERC 30.1 h post injection.

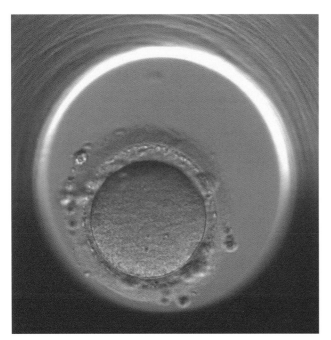

Figure 14.4 The sERC 29.4 h post injection.

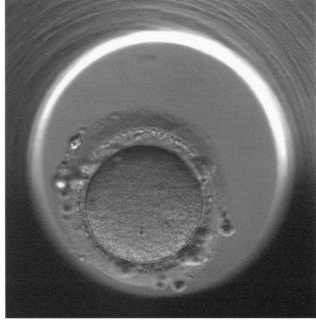

Figure 14.6 The sERC 30.6 h post injection.

oocytes should be inseminated. At CARE Fertility, sERC have been recorded, post ICSI, using the EmbryoScope time-lapse imaging system (FertiliTech, Denmark) in 0.3 percent of inseminated eggs.[6] Approximately 40 percent of these eggs fertilized normally, and three of the embryos were transferred, resulting in one healthy live birth.[6] Further studies are needed to look into the size, timing, and appearance of sERC.

Figures 14.8 and 14.9 show an oocyte with multiple sERC that went on to fertilize normally. The embryo cleaved but then fragmented and did not reach blastocyst.

REFERENCES

1. Otsuki J, Okada A, Morimoto K, et al. The relationship between pregnancy outcome and smooth endoplasmic reticulum clusters in MII oocytes. *Hum Reprod.* 2004;19: 1591–1597.
2. Sa R, Cunha M, Silva J, et al. Ultrastructure of tubular smooth endoplasmic reticulum aggregates in human metaphase II oocytes and clinical implications. *Fertil Steril.* 2011;96: 143–149.

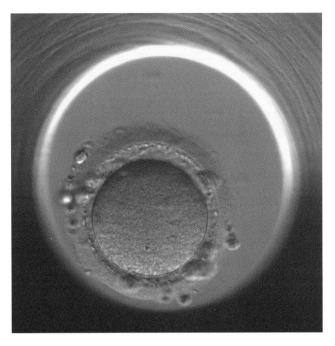

Figure 14.7 The sERC 31.3 h post injection.

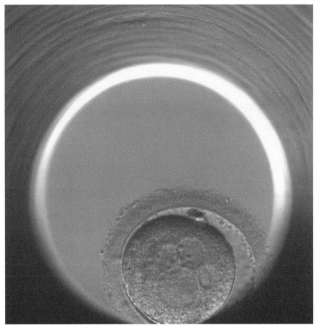

Figure 14.9 A 2PN seen with multiple sERC.

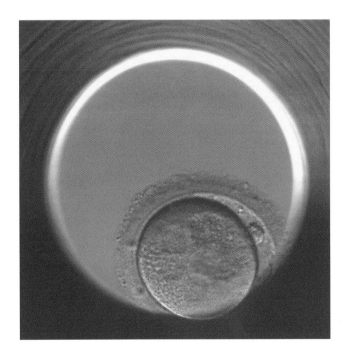

Figure 14.8 Multiple sERC seen 0.4 h post injection.

3. Miwa A, Nagai Y, Momma Y, et al. Avoiding the occurrence of smooth endoplasmic reticulum clusters in oocytes improves ART outcomes. *Hum Reprod.* 2013;28 (suppl):i184–i185.

4. Ebner T, Moser M, Shebi O, et al. Prognosis of oocytes showing aggregation of smooth endoplasmic reticulum. *Reprod Biomed Online.* 2008;16:113–118.

5. Mateizal I, Van Landuy L, Tournaye H, et al. Deliveries of normal healthy babies from embryos originating from oocytes showing the presence of smooth endoplasmic reticulum aggregates. *Hum Reprod.* 2013;28:2111–2117.

6. Campbell A, Fishel S, Cater E, et al. Retrospective assessment of time lapse data from 6730 human embryos to establish incidence rates for preimplantation cleavage anomalies. Association of Clinical Embryologists Annual Conference. January 2–4, Sheffield, 2014.

15

Multinucleation

Claire Shearer

The cell nucleus is a membrane-bound organelle containing the cell's DNA. The Istanbul Consensus Group defined *multinucleation* as the presence of more than one nucleus in a blastomere (i.e., a binary grading was proposed to note either presence or absence) and included micronuclei (ALPHA and ESHRE Interest Group of Embryology, 2011). Furthermore, multinucleation assessment was proposed to be performed ideally on day 2 (i.e., 44 ± 1 h post insemination), and the observation of multinucleation in one cell per embryo was sufficient for the embryo to be considered to be multinucleated. It was further agreed, by that special interest group, that multinucleation assessment on day 3 would be complicated by the much smaller cell size and therefore would be less reliable.[1]

As nuclei are visible only during part of the mitotic cycle, with static observations multinucleation may be missed. Multinucleation is most reliably detected by time-lapse technology.[2,3] Each blastomere should be evaluated as multinucleation may occur in one, several, or all blastomeres. Video 15.1 shows blastomeres with multinuclei developing into an irregular cleavage pattern. The video can be viewed online: http://goo.gl/vi3EMT.

The mechanisms by which multinucleated blastomeres are formed are not fully understood, and it is not clear whether multinucleated cells contain separate nuclear structures or a single nucleus that undergoes temporary changes in shape.[3] Different multinucleation phenotypes have been observed, with binucleation (i.e., two equal-sized diploid nuclei) (Figure 15.1) and micronucleation (i.e., fractured nuclei/several small nuclei which can differ in size) (Figures 15.2 to 15.5) being suggested as the two most common types.[4]

The impact of the degree and type of multinucleation has yet to be elucidated. However, Meriano et al. showed that micronucleated embryos have a higher incidence of chromosomal anomalies than binucleated embryos, and also suggested that the greater the number of cells that are multinucleated within an embryo, then the more likely the embryo is to have a poor prognosis.[4]

Multinucleation at the four-cell stage was introduced as an exclusion criterion by Meseguer and colleagues who used a hierarchical approach to embryo selection modeling. In a large, retrospective analysis of transferred embryos with known outcome, they found significant differences between implanted and not implanted embryos for six early morphokinetic variables, including multinucleation at the four-cell stage.[2] It may be conducive to annotate the different multinucleation phenotypes separately. There is published evidence that binucleated embryos may develop normally.[4,5] One study found that 30.4 percent of two-cell embryos with binucleated blastomeres progressed to entirely diploid embryos with mononucleated blastomeres.[4]

The embryo shown in Figures 15.1, 15.6 and 15.7 was transferred back into the patient along with another morula (that was multinucleated at the two-cell and four-cell stages). There was little choice for embryo transfer, and no embryos were frozen, as the whole embryo cohort for this patient exhibited multinucleation. Although both embryos implanted, the patient gave birth to only a singleton.

In light of limited data and the static-based consensus as it stands, embryos with mononucleated blastomeres should be selected preferentially where possible, especially if the multinucleation is not binucleation and is detectable beyond the two-cell stage.[1]

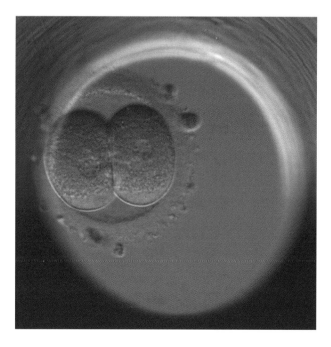

Figure 15.1 This is a two-cell embryo showing two nuclei in both cells. Binucleation can be seen clearly in the right-hand blastomere.

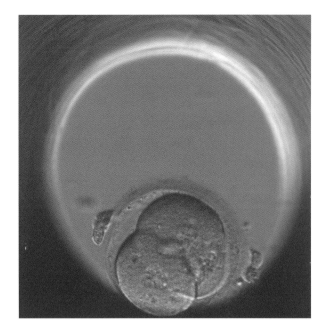

Figure 15.2 Both the cells of this two-cell embryo show multi-nucleation. Micronucleation is present in the largest of the blastomeres.

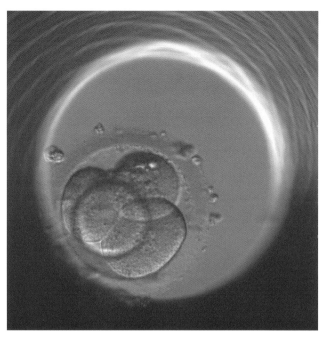

Figure 15.4 This is the same embryo as in Figure 15.3. It is at a later time point and now has four cells. Micronucleation is still present in the bottom right-hand-side blastomere.

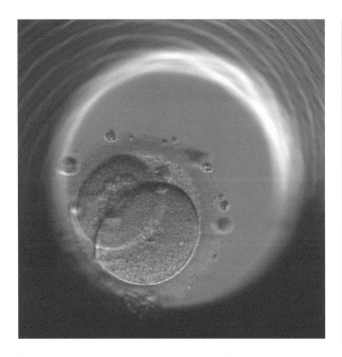

Figure 15.3 The largest blastomere of this two-cell embryo exhibits micronucleation.

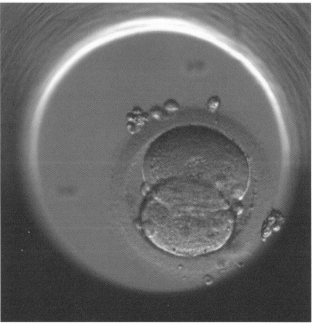

Figure 15.5 Micronucleation is present in the smaller blastomere. Two overlapping nuclei (binucleation) are visible in the other blastomere.

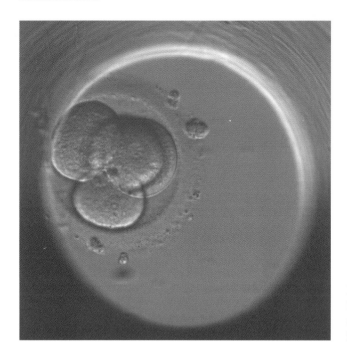

Figure 15.6 This is the same embryo that was binucleated in Figure 15.1. At 39 hours it now appears normal as it has only one nucleus in each of the four cells. This embryo developed into a good quality morula on day 4.

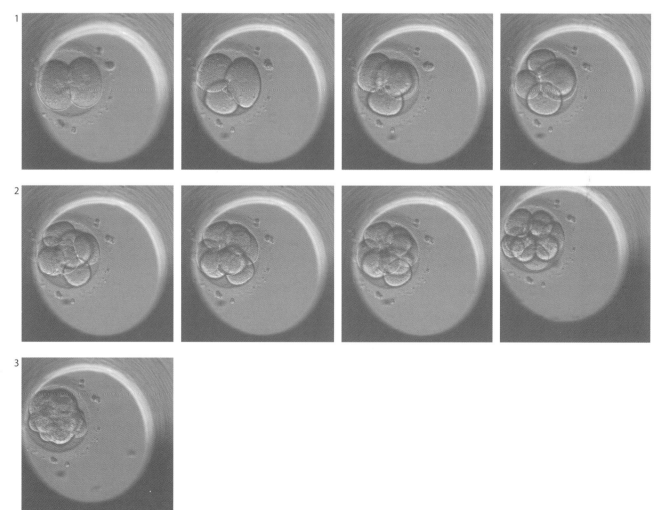

Figure 15.7 Time-lapse sequence showing this embryo's development from day 2 to day 4.

REFERENCES

1. Alpha Scientists in Reproductive Medicine and ESHRE Special Interest Group of Embryology. The Istanbul consensus workshop on embryo assessment: proceedings of an expert meeting. *Hum Reprod.* 2011;26:1270–1283.
2. Meseguer M, Herrero J, Tejera A, et al. The use of morphokinetics as a predictor of embryo implantation. *Hum Reprod.* 2011;26(10):2658–2671.
3. Ergin EG, Çökelez K. The frequency of embryo multinucleation detected by time-lapse system and its impact on pregnancy outcome. ASRM abstract. *Fertil Steril.* 2013;100(3, suppl):S69–S70.
4. Meriano J, Clark C, Cadesky K, et al. Bi-nucleated and micro-nucleated blastomeres in embryos derived from human assisted reproduction cycles. *RBM Online.* 2004;9: 511–520.
5. Staessen C, Van Steirteghem A. The genetic constitution of multinuclear blastomeres and their derivative daughter blastomeres. *Hum Reprod.* 1998;13:1625–1631.

16

Vacuolation

Rachel Smith

Vacuoles are membrane-bound, fluid-filled inclusions within the cytoplasm. They are often reported in publications as cytoplasmic inclusions, along with smooth endoplasmic reticulum (sERC) and refractile bodies, when assessing oocyte dysmorphisms. Cytoplasmic inclusions are linked to reduced fertilization and embryo development in numerous studies.[1-3] In studies where the effects of vacuoles has been investigated separately, they have been shown to be associated with a reduced incidence of fertilization, but once the oocyte is fertilized, there is no reported reduction in pronuclear or embryo morphology.[3] Vacuoles arise in different sizes and are distinguishable from other round anomalies as separated from the surrounding ooplasm by the presence of a membrane. The large vacuoles, greater in diameter than 14 um, were associated with a significant reduction in fertilization.[4] Studies examining the effects of vacuoles present in the oocyte and early embryo, and then subsequent culture to day 5, revealed no effects on blastocyst expansion and hatching.[5]

It is widely accepted that vacuoles either appear spontaneously or that they are a result of merging preexisting vesicles originating from SER and/or Golgi apparatus.[6,7] How a reduction in fertilization is caused by the presence of vacuolization is not fully understood. One suggestion is that the presence of these fluid-filled inclusions interferes with cytoskeleton function, or large vacuoles may displace the metaphase II spindle from its polar position resulting in fertilization failure.[8] Another suggestion is that their presence can affect the competence of the MII meiotic spindle.[6]

There are many different types of vacuole, not only ranging in size but in number. Three categories have been reported:

1. Those that appear during oocyte maturation and are therefore visible at oocyte collection; known as day 0.
2. Those artificially created by intracytoplasmic sperm injection (ICSI) (day 1) reported significantly higher incidence of vacuoles following ICSI ($p < 0.01$) 11.6 percent than IVF 5.3 percent[4]; and incident rates of vacuolation in oocytes from our annotations collaborate this finding ICSI ($p < 0.5$) 6.3 percent significantly higher than IVF 3.7 percent (unpublished data).
3. Those accompanied with developmental arrest (day 4). According to Ebner, the later that vacuoles appear, the more detrimental their effect on blastocyst formation. A significant reduction in blastocyst formation (p < 0.001) was demonstrated when vacuoles were present on day 4.[4]

CARE Fertility has investigated the incidence and impact of vacuolation from time-lapse images acquired by the EmbryoScope (FertiliTech, Denmark). If not already present, the time of vacuole appearance varied greatly; vacuoles first presented between 0.35 hpi and 81.4 hpi (unpublished). Of 23 transferred embryos that had vacuolation recorded as present, nine resulted in ongoing clinical pregnancy. Nevertheless, embryos resulting from oocyte with vacuolation or developing vacuolation during their in vitro development are avoided for transfer where possible. Video 16.1 shows vacuoles developing in blastomeres at 60 hpi. The video can be viewed online: http://goo.gl/bS9bkJ.

The overall incidence of vacuoles, from 11 583 time-lapse annotated 2PN embryos, was 1.2 percent. This corresponds to published incidence rates of 5.9 percent ($n = 325$) and 3.1 percent ($n = 1191$) from observed oocytes.[1,5]

Different vacuole types are seen in oocytes and zygotes. Large vacuoles present in the mature oocyte have been reported to significantly reduce fertilization[4] (Figure 16.1).

In some cases, vacuolation is present only in the early stages of development and disappears before first cleavage (Figure 16.2). This transient appearance could be missed under standard stereomicroscope assessments.

Vacuoles can be present in the oocyte and remain unchanged through to the later stages of development (Figure 16.3).

Vacuoles can appear in the oocyte and change in number through the various cleavage stages (Figure 16.4).

Vacuolation in the later cleavage stages

Figure 16.5 illustrates vacuolation in the later cleavage stages.

In the later stages of development, the formation of vacuoles is associated with degeneration. However, the late appearance of vacuolation is not always a marker for cell degeneration; Figure 16.6 shows a sequence with the vacuole first appearing at the seven-cell stage.

Vacuoles can also arise in the extracellular cytoplasm, as seen in Figure 16.7 in the polar body of a fertilized zygote.

Figure 16.8, from an abnormally fertilized zygote (3PN), outlines the devastating effect that vacuoles can have on the competency of the oocyte.

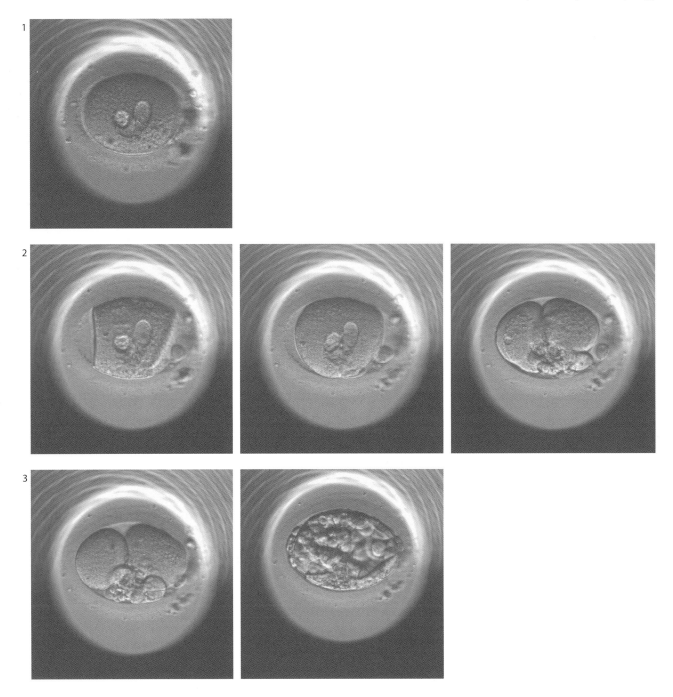

Figure 16.1 Row 1: At time 2.5 hours post insemination (hpi) following ICSI, large vacuoles greater than 14 um in diameter are present. (Left-side vacuole 26 μm × 25 μm, right-side vacuole 33 μm × 27 μm.) Row 2: 19.3 hpi: Two pronuclei visible; 23.3 hpi PN fade; 26.4 hpi two-cell division vacuoles extruded into fragments. Row 3: 36.4 hpi: Vacuoles visible in fragments, final development stage of the embryo; 113.1 hpi: Early blastocyst.

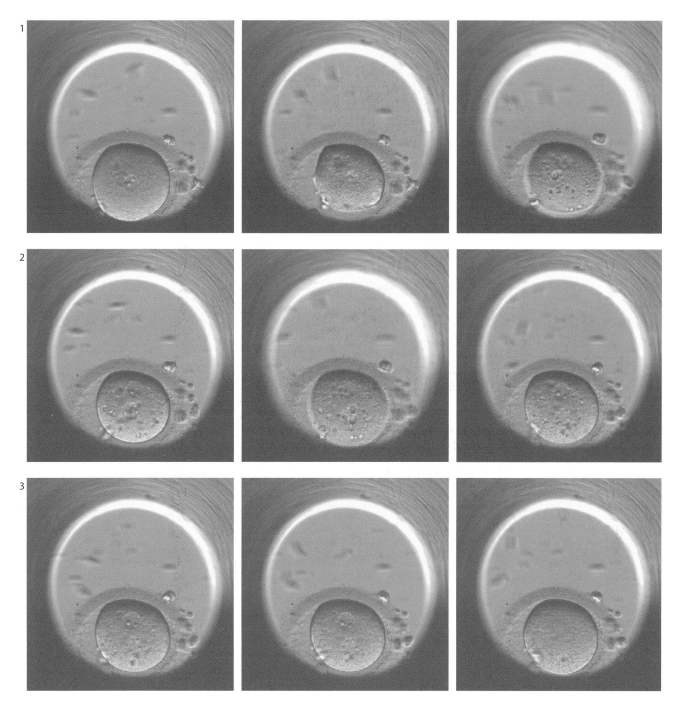

Figure 16.2 Row 1: 10.7 hpi: Normal 2PN: No vacuolation; 13.7 hpi cytoplasm constricts and shrinks; 17.4 hpi appearance of small vacuoles dispersed throughout the cytoplasm. Row 2: 18.7 hpi, 22.2 hpi, and 24.7 hpi: Multiple small vacuoles in 2PN zygote. Row 3: 26.2 hpi: Presence of vacuoles starts to decrease; 27.7 hpi only one or two vacuoles present; all have disappeared by PN fade 29 hpi

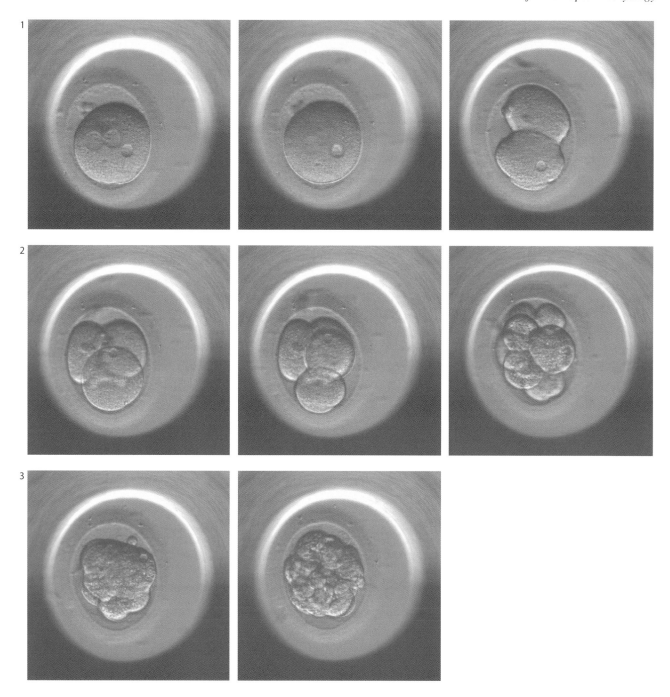

Figure 16.3 Row 1: 18.1 hpi: Single vacuole at 2PN stage, 25.6 hpi PN fade and 28.3 hpi two-cell stage. Row 2: 39.6 hpi: Single vacuole at three-cell stage, 42.4 hpi four-cell stage and 60.9 hpi at seven-cell stage. Row 3: Single vacuole still visible at morula 80.9 hpi and 96.5 hpi at start of cavitation.

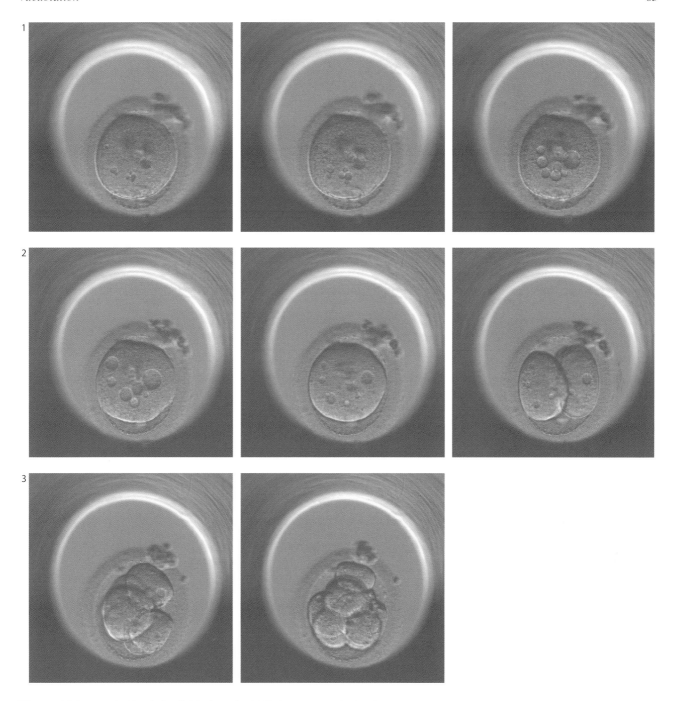

Figure 16.4 Row 1: 10.7 hpi, 12.7 hpi, and 16.4 hpi: Vacuoles in the 2PN zygote growing in size and number. Row 2: 20 hpi: Following PN fade the vacuoles start to disperse and 22.8 hpi reduce in size and number, 29 hpi fewer vacuoles visible in the two-cell embryo. Row 3: 42.8 hpi four cell and 65.9 hpi eight cell: Although size and numbers were reduced, still visible at four-cell and eight-cell stage.

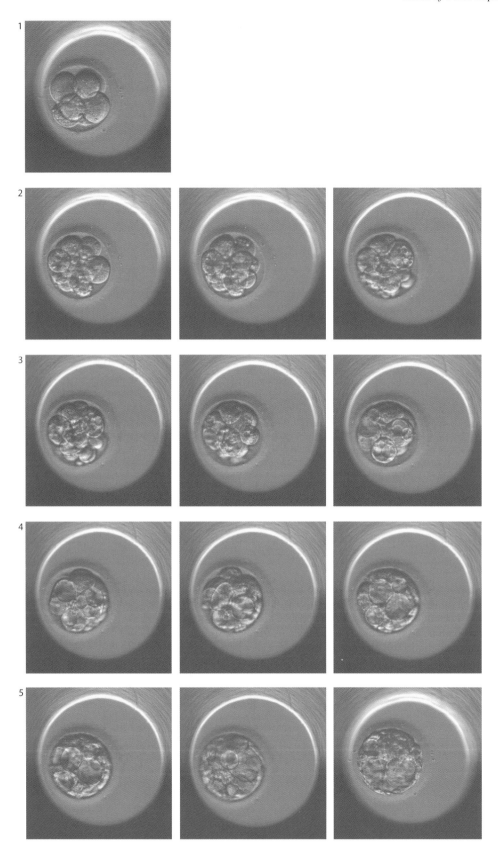

Figure 16.5 Row 1: 69.2 hpi: Seven-cell embryo, some fragmentation but no visible vacuolation, Rows 2 and 3: Growing numbers and size of vacuoles in the nine-cell embryo 81 hpi, 82.8 hpi, 83.6 hpi, 85.8 hpi, 88 hpi, and 92.3 hpi. Row 4: 97.3 hpi, 102.1 hpi, and 105.5 hpi: Large vacuoles present in the compacting morula. Row 5: 109.1 hpi, 114.5 hpi, and 120 hpi: Cavitating blastocyst has large visible vacuoles.

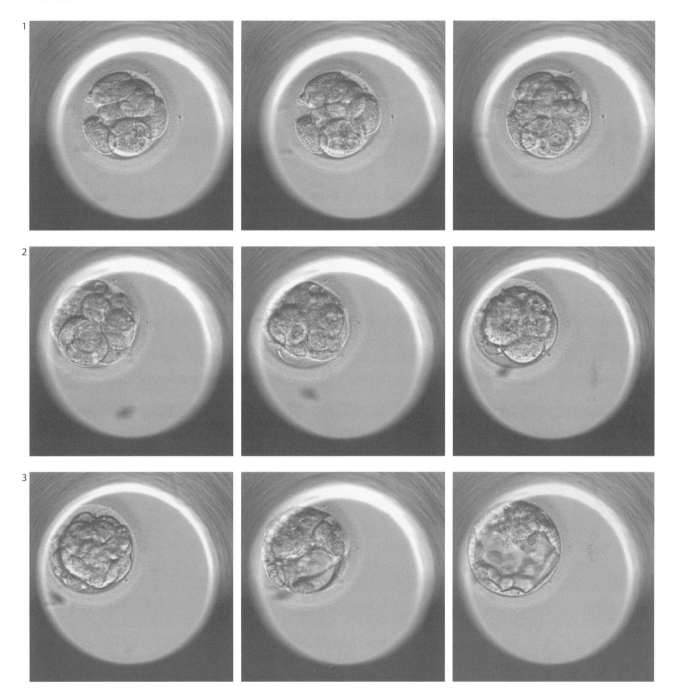

Figure 16.6 Row 1: 63.6 hpi and 66.4 hpi vacuoles present in two different cells within a seven-cell, day 3 embryo. 68 hpi still visible at the eight-cell stage. Row 2: 70.8 hpi large vacuole still visible at nine-cell stage, 75.2 hpi start of compaction vacuole looks to be extruded from the compacting morula, 79.8 hpi vacuole still visible on exterior surface of the morula. Row 3: 84.8 hpi start of cavitation vacuole still on the outer surface, 91.7 hpi cavity expanding, 96.5 hpi blastocyst with no visible vacuole.

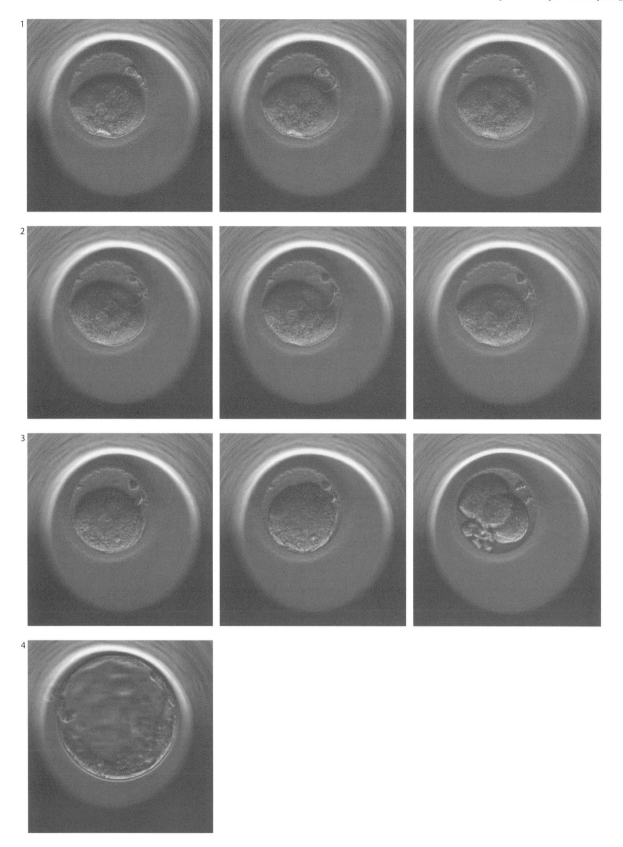

Figure 16.7 Row 1: 20.3 hpi, 22.7 hpi, and 25.9 hpi: Enlarging vacuole seen within the polar body of a 2PN stage zygote. Row 2: 28.2 hpi, 31.21 hours, and 33.7 hpi perivitelline space increases as the size of the vacuole increases to its maximum diameter. Row 3: 36.2 hpi the membrane ruptures, 39.5 hpi loss of vacuole volume and re-expansion of the ooplasm, 45.2 hpi cleavage to two cell. Row 4: Resulting stage of development, expanded blastocyst.

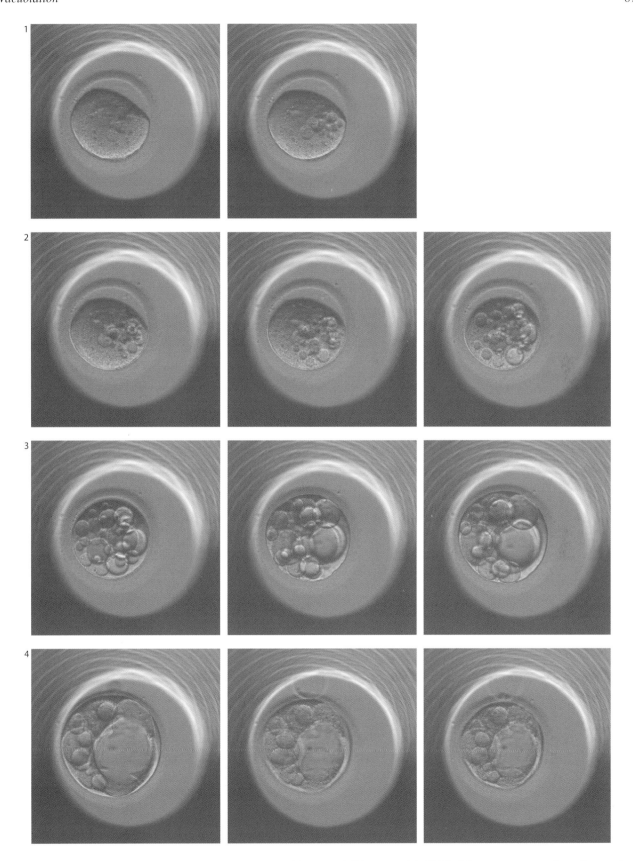

Figure 16.8 Row 1: 17 hpi abnormally fertilized oocyte with three visible pronuclei, 19.9 hpi first appearance of small vacuoles. Row 2: 22.7 hpi to 27.3 hpi the vacuoles multiply and grow in size. Row 3: 29 to 34.7 hpi the ooplasm is filled with large vacuoles which continue to change in size and number. Row 4: 38.5 hours is the start of cell death, 40.5 hpi the vacuole expansion causes a rupture in the zona, 47.7 hpi ooplasm starts to constrict as the cell degenerates.

REFERENCES

1. Renzi L, Ubaldi FM, Iacobelli M, et al. Significance of metaphase II human oocyte morphology on ICSI outcome. *Fertil Steril.* 2008;90:1692–1700.

2. Otsuki J Nagai Y, Chiba K. Lipofuscin bodies in human oocytes as an indicator of oocyte quality. *J Assist Reprod Genet.* 2007;24:263–353.

3. Xia P. Intracytoplasmic sperm injection: correlation of oocyte grade based on polar body, perivitelline space and cytoplasmic inclusions with fertilisation rate and embryo quality. *Hum Reprod.* 1997;12:1750–1755.

4. Ebner T, Moser M, Sommerguber M, et al. Occurrence and developmental consequences of vacuoles throughout preimplantation development. *Fertil Steril.* 2005;83:1635–1640.

5. Braga D, Setti A, Figueira R, et al. Influence of oocyte dysmorphisms on blastocyst formation and quality. *Fertil Steril.* 2013;100:748–753.

6. Van Blerkom J, Bell H, Weipz D. Cellular and developmental biological aspects of bovine meiotic maturation, fertilization, and preimplantation embryogenesis in vitro. *J Electron Microsc Tech.* 1990;16:298–323.

7. El Shafie M, Sousa M, Windt ML, et al. *An Atlas of the Ultrastructure of Human Oocytes: A Guide for Assisted Reproduction.* New York, NY: Parthenon; 2000:151–171.

8. Ebner T, Moser M, Tew G. Is oocyte morphology prognostic of embryo developmental potential after ICSI? *Reprod Biomed Online.* 2006;12:507–512.

17

Granular Cytoplasm

Sarah Foley

The cytoplasm of the mature human oocyte is generally uniform. Areas of irregularity in the cytoplasm, believed to be due to inclusions or clusters of organelles, are described as cytoplasmic granularity.

The causes of granulation of the oocyte cytoplasm remain unclear, although it has been postulated that it may be associated with incomplete chromosomal maturation or as a result of chromosomal abnormalities.[1] There are contradictory reports within the literature regarding the possible impact of granular cytoplasm on embryo developmental and clinical outcome. It has been reported to have no significant effect on intracytoplasmic sperm injection (ICSI) fertilization rate or embryo quality, and is not associated with reduced blastocyst development, pregnancy, or risk of miscarriage.[1–4] One study reported higher fertilization rates from ICSI oocytes displaying granulation when compared with those that did not.[5]

However, fertilization of oocytes with granular cytoplasm has also been reported to lead to poor pronuclear morphology and/or embryo quality.[6–8] In a cohort of oocytes with both normal and granular cytoplasm, the whole cohort may have a poor prognosis.[1,3] Balaban reported that embryos developed from oocytes displaying granulation had decreased survival and poor in vitro development after cryopreservation, while Kahraman et al. found no significant effect on implantation of embryos derived from granulated oocytes but the ongoing pregnancy rate was decreased.[1,9] Video 17.1 shows granulation in the zygote cytoplasm and in the developing blastomeres. The video can be viewed online: http://goo.gl/Vi5Z2j.

Granulation in the cytoplasm of an oocyte can appear throughout the oocyte (Figure 17.1) or discretely (Figure 17.2), peripherally or centrally localized.

Centrally located granulation is thought to be of more concern than the homogeneous variety, and it often appears as a dark, spongy area (Figure 17.3).[1]

The severity of the granularity is based on the size and the depth of the affected area (Figures 17.4 to 17.6).

Granular cytoplasm is predominantly described in oocytes, rather than embryos. Time-lapse imaging suggests that granulated areas are gradually dispersed throughout the ooplasm and are often not visible after the first division (Figure 17.7).

It is rarer to find granular cytoplasm in the blastomeres of cleavage-stage embryos (Figure 17.8).

When granulation is seen in either oocytes or embryos during the annotation process, then it is entered into the comments section for that particular embryo. The incidence of granulation across CARE units appears very small with only 10 reported

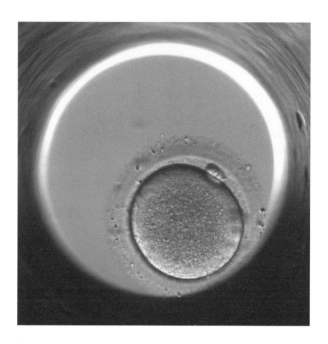

Figure 17.1 Localized granulation.

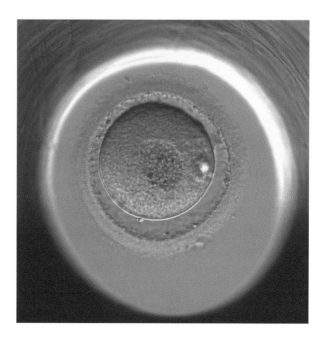

Figure 17.2 Central granulation.

(a)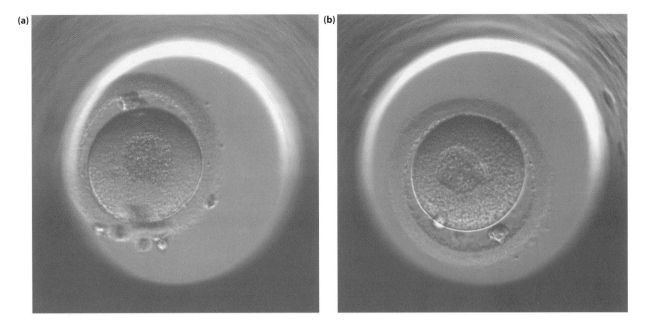(b)

Figure 17.3 Central granulation.

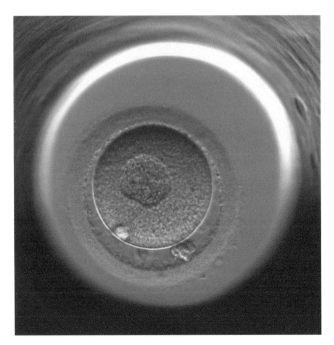

Figure 17.4 Severe localized granulation.

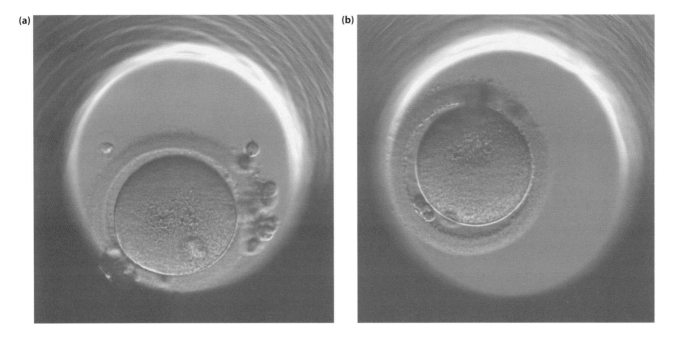

Figure 17.5 (a) Fine central granulation. (b) Fine centrally localized granulation.

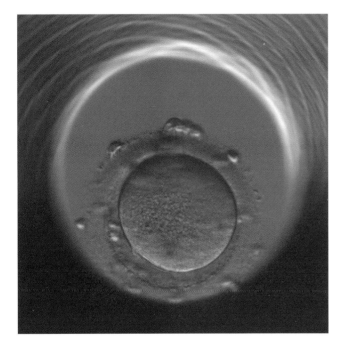

Figure 17.6 Dispersed fine granulation.

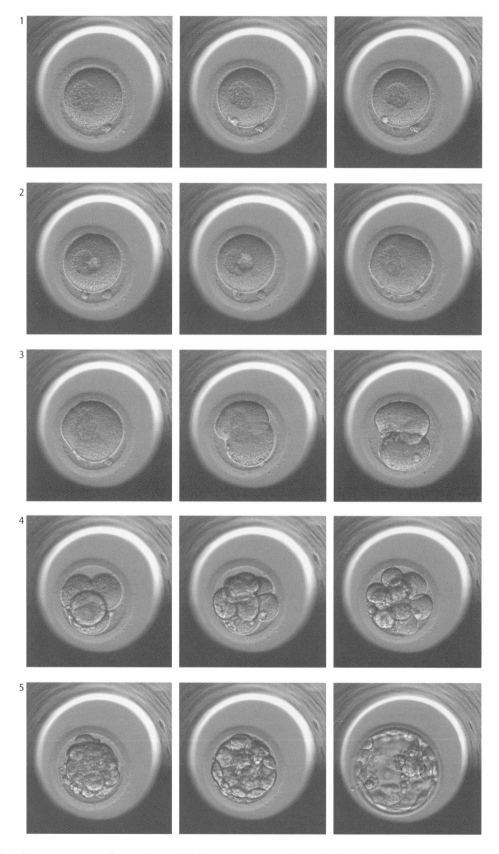

Figure 17.7 Development pattern of an embryo exhibiting severe central granulation (rows 1 to 3, up to the first cleavage, row 4 from 4 to 10 cells and row 5, compaction to expansion).

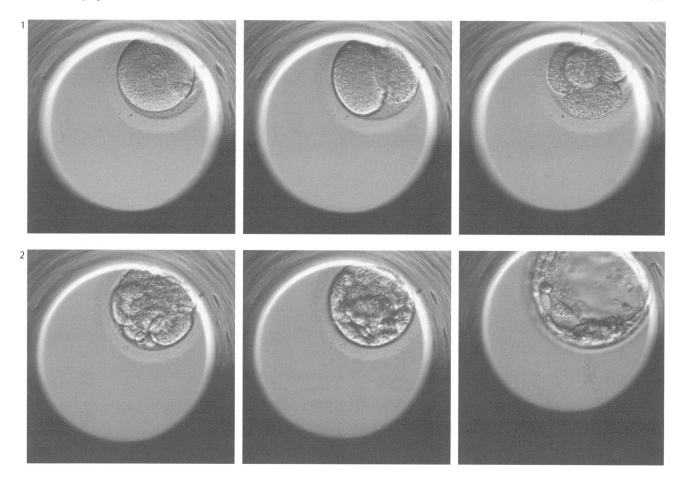

Figure 17.8 Granular cytoplasm within an embryo. Series of images demonstrating development to blastocyst.

cases, and only one of these embryos has been transferred which did not lead to a pregnancy.

REFERENCES

1. Kahraman S, Yakin K, Donmez E, et al. Relationship between granular cytoplasm of oocytes and pregnancy outcome following intracytoplasmic sperm injection. *Hum Reprod.* 2000;15:2390–2393.
2. Serhal PF, Ranieri DM, Kinis A, et al. Oocyte morphology predicts outcome of intracytoplasmic sperm injection. *Hum Reprod.* 1997;12:1267–1270.
3. Meriano JS, Alexis J, Visram-Zaver S, et al. Tracking of oocyte dysmorphisms for ICSI patients may prove relevant to the outcome in subsequent patient cycles. *Hum Reprod.* 2001;16(10):2118–2123.
4. Braga D, Setti A, de Cássia R, et al. Influence of oocyte dysmorphisms on blastocyst formation and quality. *Fertil Steril.* 2013;3:748–754.
5. Wilding M, Di ML, D'Andretti S, et al. An oocyte score for use in assisted reproduction. *J Assist Reprod Genet.* 2007;24:350–358.
6. Loutradis D, Drakakis P, Kallianidis K, et al. Oocyte morphology correlates with embryo quality and pregnancy rate after intracytoplasmic sperm injection. *Fertil Steril.* 1999;72:240–244.
7. Ten J, Mendiola J, Vioque J, et al. Donor oocyte dysmorphisms and their influence on fertilization and embryo quality. *Reprod Biomed Online.* 2007;14:40–48.
8. Rienzi L, Ubaldi FM, Iacobelli M, et al. Significance of metaphase II human oocyte morphology on ICSI outcome. *Fertil Steril.* 2008;90:1692–1700.
9. Balaban B, Ata B, Isiklar A, et al. Severe cytoplasmic abnormalities of the oocyte decrease cryosurvival and subsequent embryonic development of cryopreserved embryos. *Hum Reprod.* 2008;23:1778–1785.

18

Zona Defects

Gerri Emerson

The zona pellucida (ZP) surrounding the mammalian oocyte is a translucent glycoproteinaceous matrix and has a critical role to play in oogenesis, fertilization (by acting as a 'docking site' for the binding of spermatozoa), and induction of the acrosome reaction of spermatozoa that attach.[1] Its thickness and protein content can vary considerably between species (1 to 25 μm).[2] In humans the ZP matrix is composed of four glycoproteins, designated as ZP1, ZP2, ZP3, ZP4, instead of three found in the commonly studied mouse ZP. The zona proteins possess the archetypal *ZP domain*, a signature domain composed of approximately 260 amino acid residues.[3] It has been demonstrated the ZP1, ZP3 and ZP4 bind to the capacitated human spermatozoa and induce an acrosome reaction, whereas in mice, ZP3 acts as the putative primary sperm receptor. Human ZP2 binds only to acrosome-reacted spermatozoa and thus may be acting as a secondary sperm receptor.[4]

Zona Pellucida Glycoprotein 1

Zona pellucida glycoprotein 1 (ZP1) is a 638 amino acid glycoprotein located in the zona pellucida. It is synthesized by and surrounding the oocyte. The ZP1 is the least abundant glycoprotein of the four in both humans and mouse oocytes. However, despite its low abundance, it is essential for the structural integrity of the zona matrix in mice.[4,5]

Zona Pellucida Glycoprotein 2

Zona pellucida glycoprotein 2 (ZP2) is a 745 amino acid glycoprotein located in the zona pellucida, synthesized by and surrounding the oocyte. The protein acts as a secondary sperm receptor that binds sperm only after the induction of the sperm acrosome reaction. Before fertilization ZP2 binds spermatozoa. After fertilization ZP2 is proteolytically cleaved as an initial block to polyspermy.[5]

Zona Pellucida Glycoprotein 3

Zona pellucida glycoprotein 3 (ZP3) is a 424 amino acid glycoprotein located in the zona pellucida. It is synthesized by and surrounding the oocyte required for initial zona matrix formation and during fertilization for species-specific sperm binding. It is now thought to exist in two isoforms ZP3A and ZP3B (a second polymorphic allele).[5]

Zona Pellucida Glycoprotein 4

Zona pellucida glycoprotein 4 (ZP4) is a 540 amino acid glycoprotein located in the zona pellucida. It is synthesized by and surrounding the oocyte required for initial zona matrix formation and along with ZP3 during fertilization for inducing the acrosome reaction and inhibiting the binding of spermatozoa to zona pellucida in a time- and dose-dependent reaction.[5]

Zona Pellucida Binding Protein

Zona pellucida binding protein (ZPBP) is not a zona pellucida protein, but a spermatozoan protein found on the acrosome surface and one of several proteins that participate in secondary binding between acrosome-reacted spermatozoa and the zona pellucida.[5]

Zona Pellucida Birefringence

Zona pellucida birefringence (ZPB) is defined as the double refraction of light in a transparent, molecularly ordered material, which is manifested by the existence of orientation-dependent differences in the refractive index. The ZPB is the optical property of the zona pellucida using polarization imaging when viewed microscopically. This property has been used to qualitatively predict the developmental potential of in vitro matured metaphase-II (MII) oocytes.

High birefringence, compared to low, has been associated with oocytes contributing to conception cycles when compared with those of nonconception cycles and higher implantation, pregnancy, and live birth rates from transferred oocytes.[6,7] This work continues from the earlier discovery of an increased birefringence in the meiotic spindle, an early indicator of oocyte activation.[8]

Zona Pellucida Birefringence in In Vivo and In Vitro Matured Oocytes

In 2010, Daniela Paes de Almeida Ferreira Braga and colleagues reported that among immature oocytes, an increased percentage of high birefringence in prophase-I stage oocytes compared to metaphase-I stage oocytes was observed (50.7 versus 25 percent). However, the percentage of oocytes with high birefringence recorded did not change when comparing oocytes before and after in vitro maturation for both prophase-I and metaphase-I oocytes. No influence of ZPB was observed on the spontaneous in vitro maturation potential. Exclusively for metaphase II retrieved oocytes, a positive influence of ZPB on fertilization (odds ratio [OR], 1.78; 95 percent confidence interval [CI], 1.27 to 2.49) and embryo quality (OR, 2.28; 95 percent CI, 1.04 to 4.99) was noted.[7]

Zona Pellucida Anomalies and Causes

After fertilization, the zona plays a role in blocking polyspermic fertilization; it protects the integrity of the preimplantation embryo during early embryonic development and also helps its oviductal transport. Zona hardening (when a protease released from the cortical granules partially hydrolyses the zona pellucida glycoproteins, ZP2 and ZP3, removing sperm-binding capacity but also leading to a general hardening of the zona pellucida[9]) occurs naturally after fertilization in order to ensure this threefold function. A combination of lysins, produced by the cleaving embryo or the uterus, and physical expansion then reduce the zona thickness in preparation for hatching.[10] However, zona hardening is not readily quantifiable and may also be induced by prolonged exposure of oocytes and embryos to artificial culture conditions such as those in in vitro fertilization. Both maternal age and controlled ovarian stimulation regimes have been reported as contributors to zona hardening and other zonal defects such as zona thickness and density.[11] Nonspherical shapes of oocytes/embryos, within a spherical zona, have been noted in oocytes retrieved from ovaries after controlled stimulation. The causative factors remain unknown, and most probably are a product of the oocyte retrieval procedure. Likewise, nonspherical zonae are observed and appear to be the cause of nonspherical oocyte morphology within. Measuring tools within the software of time-lapse devices may be used to record the depth of the zona pellucida. Figure 18.1 and Video 18.1 were acquired using EmbryoScope™ (FertiliTech, Denmark), and the sizes reported demonstrate how the measurements of the zona pellucida can alter during embryo development due to the structure and nature of it and the movement and number of cells within it. Of course, the zona pellucida is not precisely uniform, and measurements can differ according to the specific site measured (Figure 18.1). Video 18.1 shows development of an embryo with an atypical zona pellucida. The video can be viewed online: http://goo.gl/v3Upd7.

Effects of Zona Anomalies on Fertilization, Embryo Development, and Implantation

Defective sperm-zona pellucida binding and penetration are the main causes of in vitro fertilization (IVF) failure. Animal studies undertaken to evaluate the effect of zona pellucida thickness in fertilization failure and test the influence of zona pellucida thickness on implantation and birth have shown that zona pellucida thickness has an important influence on in vivo fertilization and implantation processes but not on birth.[12] In human studies, changes in zona thickness correlated with the number of blastomeres, grade, fragmentation, and age, and were more evident in embryos transferred from cycles resulting in successful pregnancies.[13]

A meta-analysis undertaken in 2011 on the effects of oocyte morphological abnormalities on intracytoplasmic sperm injection (ICSI) outcomes, showed no reduction in fertilization or embryo development that could be attributed to zona pellucida anomalies.[14] However, in an earlier study it was postulated that resulting embryos may have a reduced potential for implantation and further development.[15] Of note, these studies were undertaken on cohorts of ICSI oocytes; therefore, as ICSI bypasses any possible zona defects, these studies only prove the effectiveness of ICSI when dealing with zona pellucida factors (Figures 18.2 to 18.19).

Conclusion

Continuous monitoring of zona pellucida characteristics of human oocytes and their resulting embryos by time lapse has enabled us to follow more closely developmental changes that occur during culture. The time-lapse images presented in this chapter show zona defects during the development of the oocyte from fertilization through to the hatching blastocyst. However, in relation to the zona pellucida, zona thinning or lack of such is not the only indicator of an embryo's potential to implant. Finally, there are many markers of oocyte functionality continuously being investigated such as cumulus, polar body, cytoplasm, and zona pellucida. However, no single characteristic has been infallible in predicting the ability of the oocyte to achieve a pregnancy. Hence, research to identify reliable markers for the assessment of oocyte quality remains a priority.

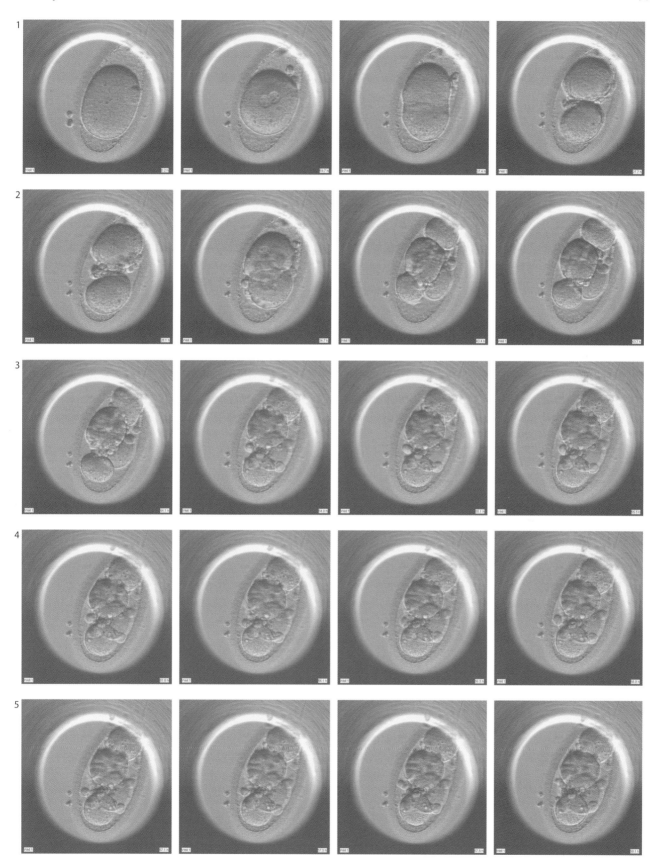

Figure 18.1 Series of time-lapse images showing the development of a nonspherical embryo. The ZP remains nonspherical throughout the cell divisions. (Timings: row 1, panel 1, 0.2 h; row 2, panel 1, 28.1 h; row 3, panel 1, 44.1 h; row 4, panel 1, 55.8 h; row 5, panel 1, 57.1 h; row 6, panel 1, 58.5 h; row 7, panel 1, 59.8 h; row 8, panel 1, 64.8 h; row 9, panel 1, 66.2 h.)

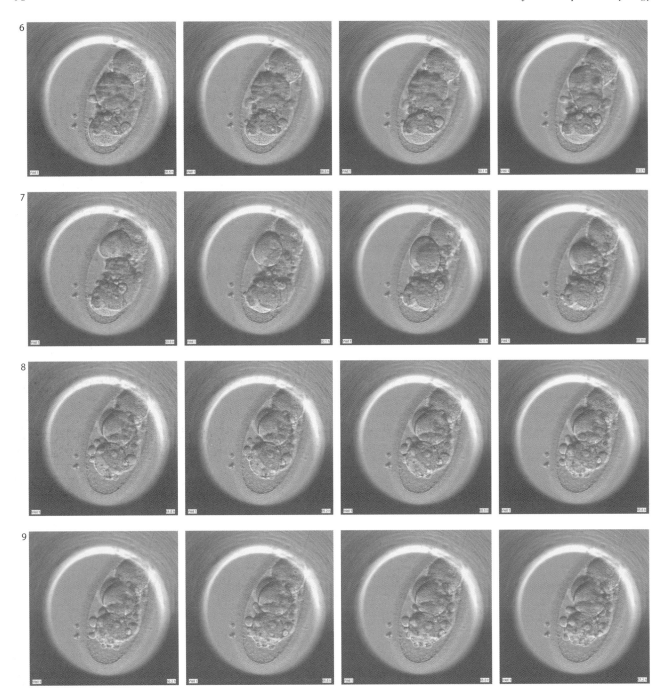

Figure 18.1 (Continued)

(a)

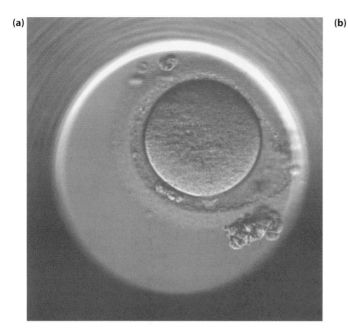

(b)

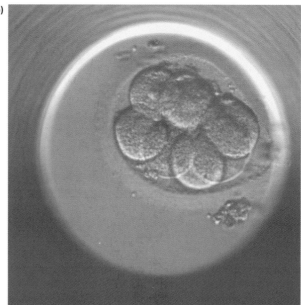

(c)

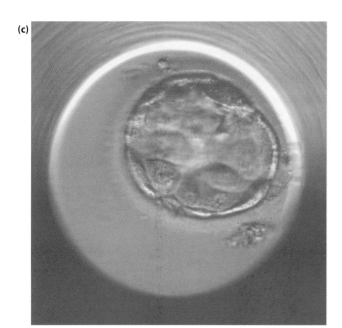

Figure 18.2 Oocyte collected from a 37-year-old woman who had undergone IVF. (a) Zona was nonspherical in appearance and measured 18 μm at 2.4 hours post insemination (hpi). (b) At the eight-cell stage (65.6 hpi) the zona measured 18 μm (no thinning). (c) At the blastocyst stage (114.6 hours) the zona measured 17 μm. This blastocyst was deemed suitable for vitrification and following warming resulted in a positive pregnancy test.

(a)

(b)

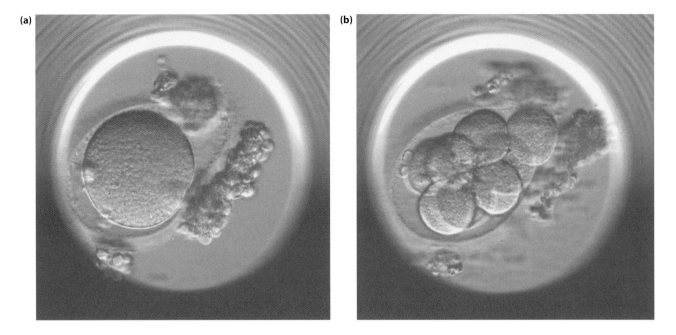

(c)

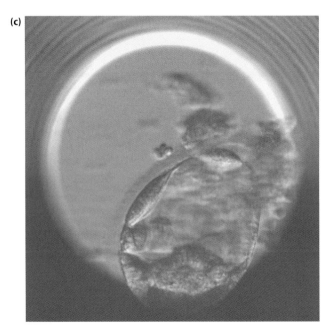

Figure 18.3 Oocyte collected from a 37-year-old woman who had undergone IVF: (a) 2.9 hpi, (b) at eight-cell stage, 44.7 hpi. The zona was nonspherical in appearance and varied in measurement from 12 to 14 μm. (c) At the blastocyst stage (93.8 hpi) the zona measured 10 to 14 μm. This blastocyst was deemed suitable for vitrification.

(a)

(b)

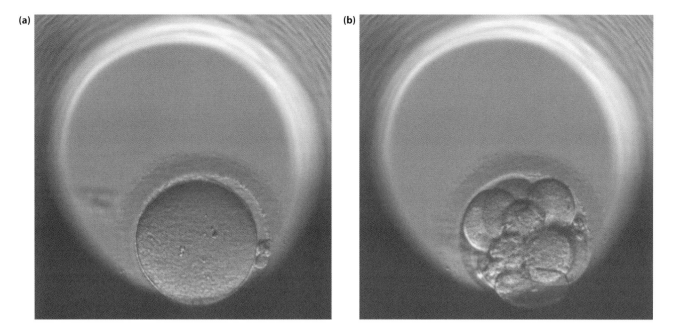

(c)

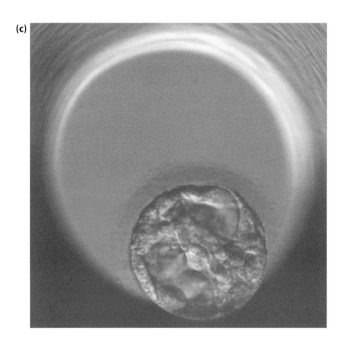

Figure 18.4 Oocyte collected from a 36-year-old woman who had undergone IVF. (a) Zona measurement at 1.6 hpi was 20 μm and (b) at 45.9 hpi (eight-cell stage) the zona measured 20 μm. (c) At the blastocyst stage (93 hpi) the zona measured 18 μm. Following transfer, the pregnancy test was negative.

(a)

(b)

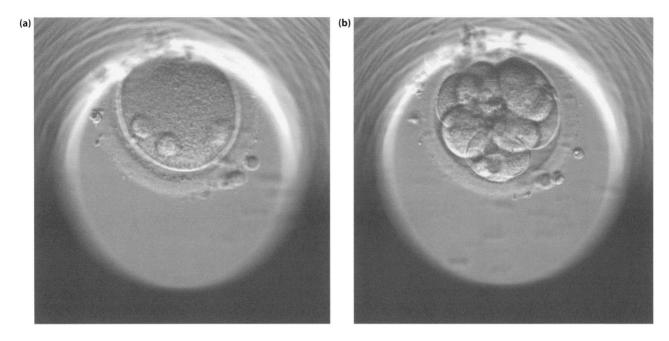

(c)

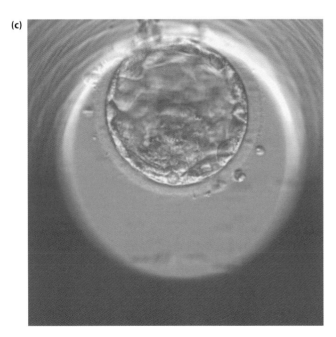

Figure 18.5 Oocyte collected from a 37-year-old woman who had undergone IVF. (a) Zona measurement at 3 hpi was 16 μm. (b) At eight-cell stage (55.3 hpi) it showed zona measurement of 16 μm. (c) At the blastocyst stage (106.6 hpi), the zona measured 12 μm. This blastocyst was vitrified/warmed and implanted resulting in a positive fetal heart and ongoing pregnancy.

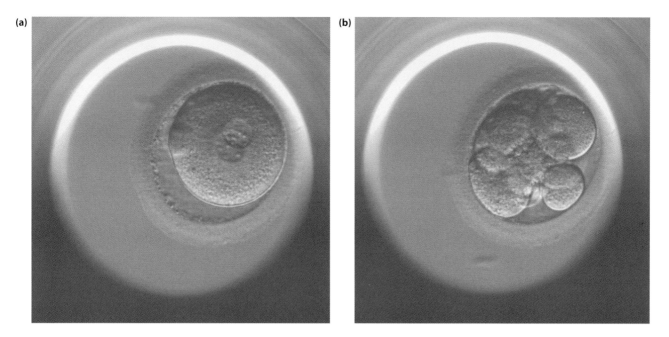

Figure 18.6 Oocyte collected from a 39-year-old woman who had undergone IVF. (a) Zona measurement at 19.2 hpi was 20 µm. (b) At eight-cell stage (49 hpi), zona measured 19 µm. Following transfer, the pregnancy test was negative.

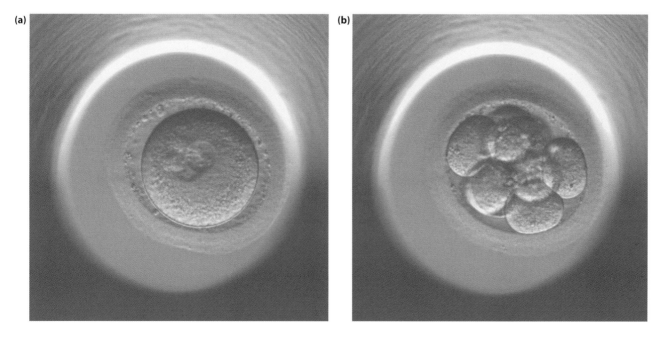

Figure 18.7 Oocyte collected from a 39-year-old woman who had undergone IVF. (a) Zona measurement at 19.2 hpi was 19 µm. (b) At eight-cell stage (50.8 hpi), zona measured 20 µm. Following transfer, the pregnancy test was negative.

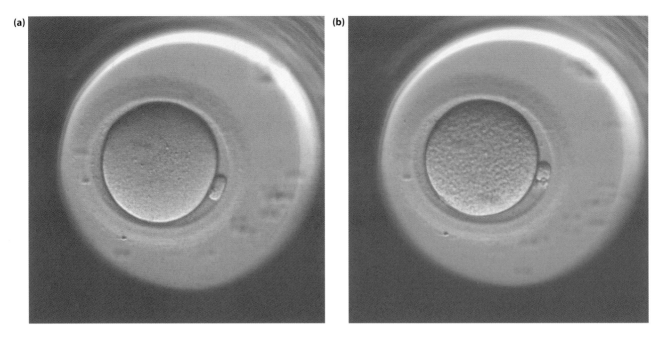

Figure 18.8 Oocyte collected from a 31-year-old woman. All oocytes failed to fertilize by IVF. Poor sperm binding was present (only one sperm in zona matrix). (a) Zona measured 21 μm at 24 hpi of culture. (b) At 115.9 hpi, it also measured 21 μm. Zona appears to have defined layers.

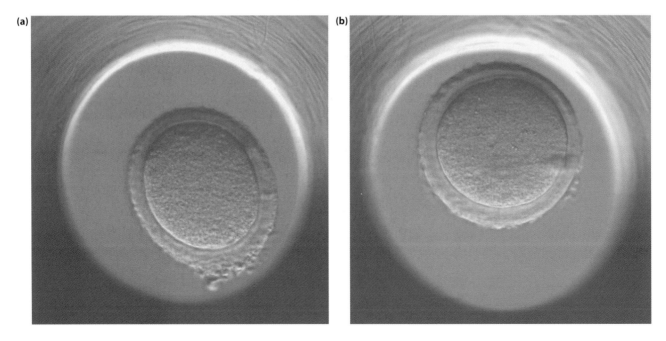

Figure 18.9 Oocytes collected from a 35-year-old woman who had undergone IVF. All oocytes and zona had a degenerate appearance.

(a)

(b)

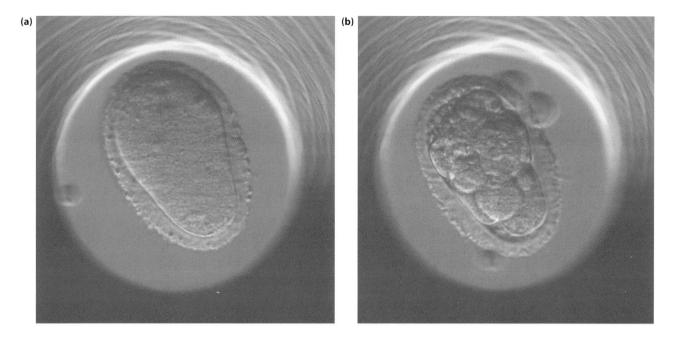

(c)

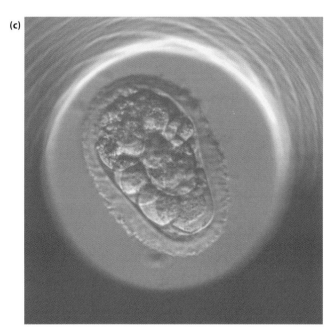

Figure 18.10 (a) Oocyte zona varied in thickness from 10 to 16 μm at 0.5 hpi of culture. (b) At 64.1 hpi, zona thickness measured 13 to 17 μm. (c) At 145.3 hpi, zona measured 13 to 16 μm. This patient had nothing suitable for transfer.

(a)   (b)

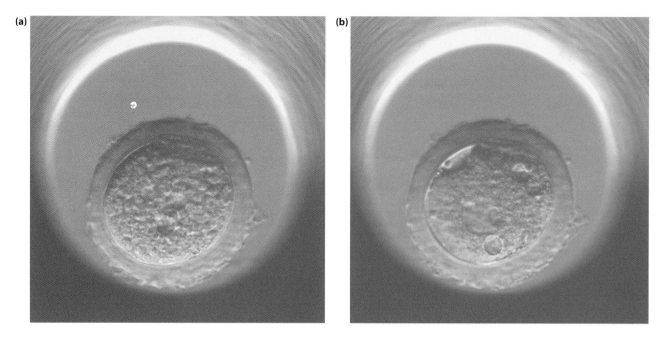

Figure 18.11 Oocyte collected from a 35-year-old woman who had undergone IVF. Zona appeared degenerative at (a) 0.5 hpi and (b) 135.5 hpi. No fertilization from ICSI.

(a)

(b)

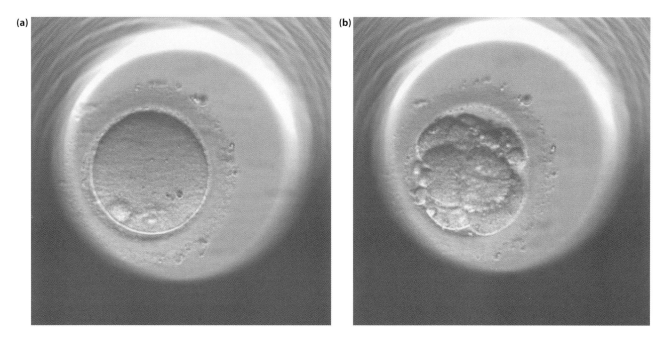

(c)

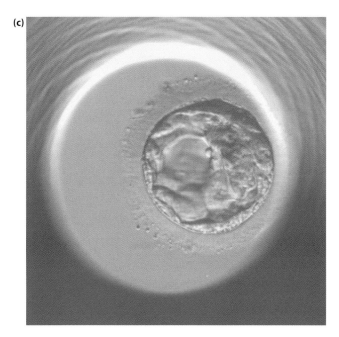

Figure 18.12 Oocyte collected from a 35-year-old woman who had undergone IVF. (a) Zona measurement at 1.8 hpi was 24 μm. (b) At eight-cell stage (55.7 hpi), it showed zona measurement of 20 μm. (c) At blastocyst (97.6 hpi) the zona measured 17 μm. The blastocyst was transferred and implanted resulting in a positive fetal heart.

(a)

(b)

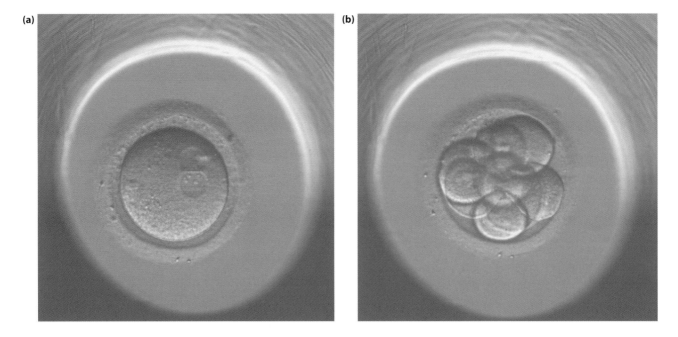

(c)

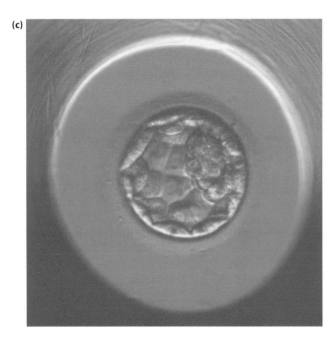

Figure 18.13 Oocyte collected from a 37-year-old woman who had undergone IVF. (a) Zona measurement at 20.3 hpi was 13 μm. (b) At eight-cell stage (51.5 hpi) it showed zona measurement of 11 μm. (c) At blastocyst (106.1 hpi), the zona measured 10 μm. Blastocyst was transferred and implanted resulting in a positive fetal heart.

(a)

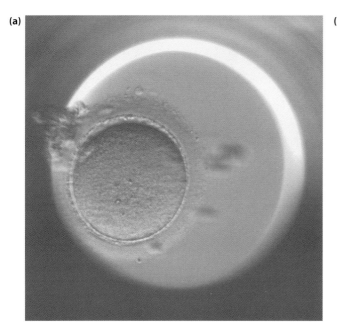

(b)

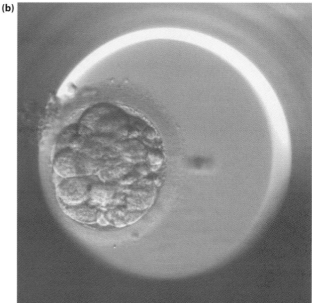

(c)

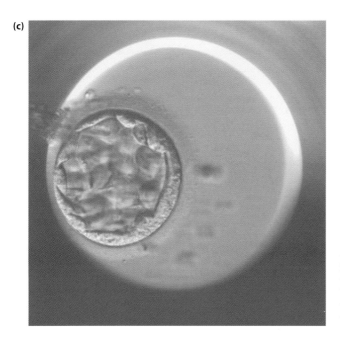

Figure 18.14 Oocyte collected from a 33-year-old woman who had undergone IVF. (a) Zona measured 17 μm at 1.1 hpi. (b) At the eight-cell stage (56.6 hpi) the zona measured 16 μm. (c) At the blastocyst stage (115.5 hpi) the zona measured 13 μm. This blastocyst was transferred but the pregnancy test was negative.

(a)

(b)

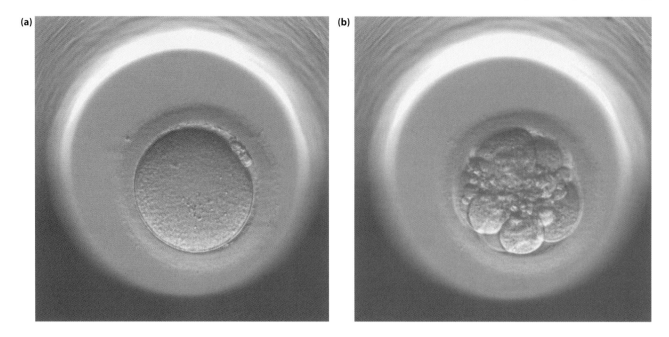

(c)

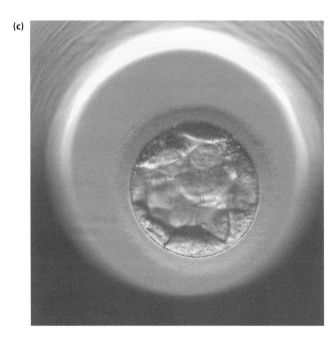

Figure 18.15 Oocyte collected from a 33-year-old woman who had undergone IVF. (a) Zona measured 20 μm at 0.4 hpi. (b) At the eight-cell stage (67.5 hpi) the zona measured 18 μm. (c) At the blastocyst stage (115.5 hpi) the zona measured 17 μm. This blastocyst was transferred but the pregnancy test was negative.

(a)

(b)

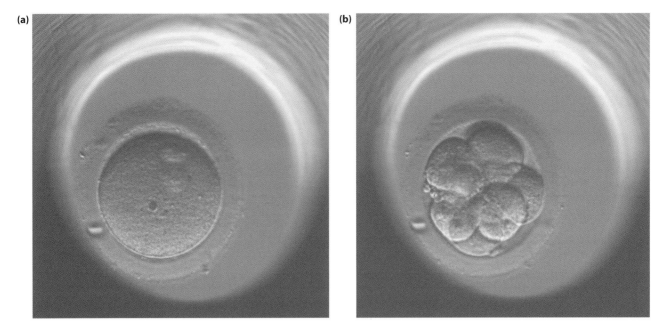

(c)

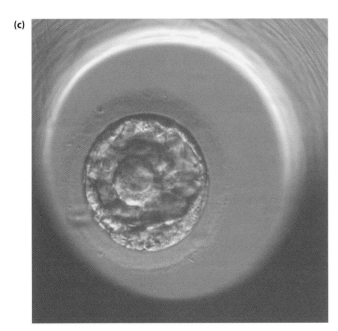

Figure 18.16 Oocyte collected from a 32-year-old woman who had undergone IVF. (a) Zona measured 17 μm at 1.7 hpi. (b) At the eight-cell stage (47.6 hpi) the zona measured 17 μm. (c) At the blastocyst stage (105.5 hpi) the zona measured 18 μm. This blastocyst was transferred and resulted in a positive fetal heart.

(a)

(b)

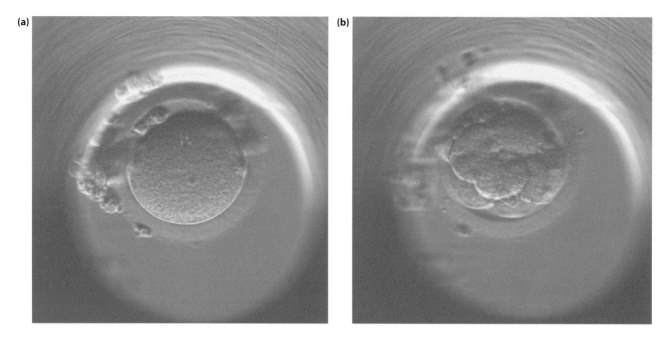

(c)

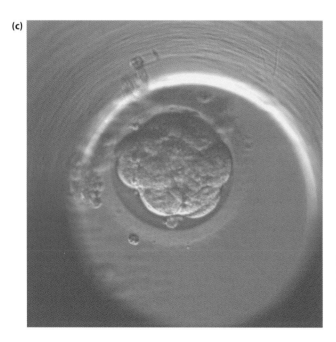

Figure 18.17 Oocyte collected from a 33-year-old woman who had undergone IVF. (a) Zona measured 13 μm at 1.2 hpi. (b) At the eight-cell stage (52.7 hpi) the zona measured 16 μm. (c) At the morula stage (91.3 hpi) the zona measured 14 μm. This morula was transferred but the pregnancy test was negative.

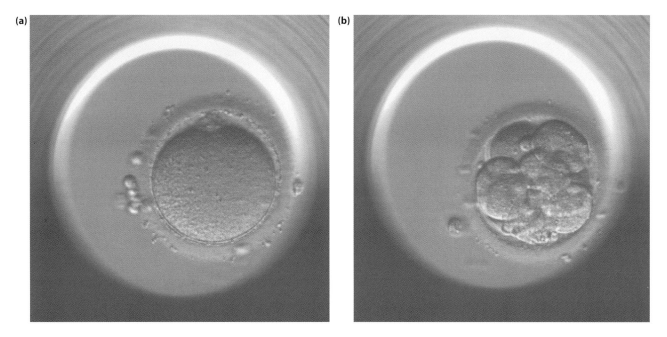

Figure 18.18 This oocyte was collected from a 35-year-old woman who had undergone IVF. (a) Zona measured 14 μm at 0.2 hpi. (b) At the eight-cell stage (62.5 hpi) the zona measured 13 μm. This embryo was transferred and resulted in a positive fetal heart.

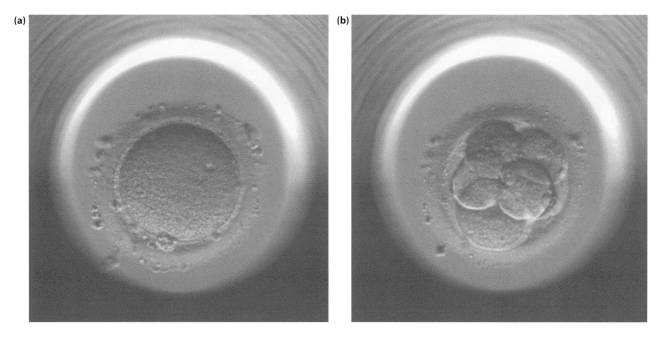

Figure 18.19 Oocyte was collected from a 35-year-old woman who had undergone IVF. (a) Zona measured 16 μm at 0.2 hpi. (b) At the eight-cell stage (59.6 hpi) the zona measured 16 μm. This embryo was transferred and resulted in a positive fetal heart.

REFERENCES

1. Gupta SK, Chakravarty S, Suraj K, et al. Structural and functional attributes of zona pellucida glycoproteins. *Soc Reprod Fertil* 2007;63(suppl):203–216.
2. Wassarman PM. Zona pellucida glycoproteins. *J Biol Chem.* 2008;283:24285–24289.
3. Ganguly A, Bansal P, Gupta T, et al. "ZP domain" of human zona pellucida glycoprotein-1 binds to human spermatozoa and induces acrosomal exocytosis. *Reprod Biol Endocrinol.* 2010 Sep 11;8:110.
4. Gupta SK, Bhandari B, Shrestha A, et al. Mammalian zona pellucida glycoproteins: structure and function during fertilization. *Cell Tissue Res.* 2012 Sep;349(3):665–678.
5. Online Mendelian Inheritance in Man®. (OMIM), a knowledgebase of human genes and genetic disorders. Nucleic Acids Research. 2005;33(suppl 1):D515–D517.
6. Montag M, Schimming T, Köster M, et al. Oocyte zona birefringence intensity is associated with embryonic implantation potential in ICSI cycles. *Reprod Biomed Online.* 2008;16(2):239–244.
7. Paes de Almeida Ferreira Braga D, de Cássia Savio Figueira R, Queiroz P, et al. Zona pellucida birefringence in in vivo and in vitro matured oocytes. *Fertil Steril.* 2010;94(6):2050–2053.
8. Liu L, Trimarchi JR, Oldenbourg R, et al. Increased birefringence in the meiotic spindle provides a new marker for the onset of activation in living oocytes. *Biol Reprod.* 2000; 63(1):251–258.
9. Dale B, De Felice L. Polyspermy prevention: facts and artefacts? *J Assist Reprod Genet.* 2011;28:199–207.
10. De Vos A, Van Steirteghem A. Zona hardening, zona drilling and assisted hatching: new achievements in assisted reproduction. *Cells Tissues Organs.* 2000;166(2):220–227.
11. Kilani SS, Cooke S, Kan AK, et al. Do age and extended culture affect the architecture of the zona pellucida of human oocytes and embryos? *Zygote.* 2006 Feb;14(1):39–44.
12. Marco-Jimenez F, Naturil-Alfonso C, Jimenez-Trigos E, et al. Influence of zona pellucida thickness on fertilization, embryo implantation and birth. *Anim Reprod Sci.* 2012 May;132(1–2):96–100.
13. Garside WT, Loret de Mola JR, Bucci JA, et al. Sequential analysis of zona thickness during in vitro culture of human zygotes: correlation with embryo quality, age, and implantation. *Mol Reprod Dev.* 1997 May;47(1):99–104.
14. Setti AS, Figueira RC, Braga DP. Relationship between oocyte abnormal morphology and intracytoplasmic sperm injection outcomes: a meta-analysis. *Eur J Obstet Gynecol Reprod Biol.* 2011 Dec;159(2):364–370.
15. Alikani M, Palermo G, Adler A. Intracytoplasmic sperm injection in dysmorphic human oocytes. *Zygote.* 1995 Nov;3(4):283–288.

19

The Patient Perspective

Samantha Duffy

CARE Fertility was the first centre in the United Kingdom to implement time-lapse microscopy as a clinical tool for embryo evaluation and selection, and the first to publish a link between morphokinetics and blastocyst ploidy.[1] Analysis of the time-lapse data has led to an increased understanding of embryo morphokinetics and the development of centre-specific selection models. Embryologists now apply this knowledge to enhance the prediction of the embryo with the highest implantation potential.[1]

The first UK IVF live birth from the use of EmbryoScope (FertiliTech, Denmark) for clinical time-lapse monitoring of embryos occurred at CARE Fertility Manchester in February 2012. Since then the use of time-lapse microscopy in patient treatment cycles has become an option at all CARE Fertility units throughout the United Kingdom and Ireland. CARE-specific predictive algorithms using EmbryoScope for time-lapse image acquisition and data collection are offered as 'CAREmaps' to patients. 'Maps' is an acronym for 'morphokinetic algorithms to predict success,' and relative uplifts in clinical outcome have been achieved using this methodology when comparing clinical results with embryos cultured and selected using standard methodology (unpublished).

As part of CAREmaps, patients can choose to receive time-lapse video footage of the embryo(s) they have transferred back during their IVF treatment. Patients receive a web link via e-mail to an in house–developed online patient area. The software generates a patient-specific PIN code to enable images to be downloaded by the patients and saved for future viewing, thus enabling them to have their very first "baby picture."

At many IVF units the traditional method of enabling patients to view their embryo(s), via a monitor in the embryo transfer room, is employed. Before the embryos are loaded into the catheter for the transfer procedure, the embryologist will focus in on the embryos in the culture dish, and the patients will be able to view them in real time on the monitor. Some units also provide patients with a printed photograph of their embryo(s) to take home.

The approach by CARE to enable patients to download and save time-lapse images was a novel one and thus was introduced following detailed consideration and was monitored closely. As part of the patient online area, an electronic questionnaire was created to encourage patient feedback that was quick and easy to complete and would give CARE an opportunity to monitor the uptake of this facility and improve the service for future treatment cycles.

The questionnaire contains six questions with set responses ranging from strongly agree to strongly disagree. An option to leave free text comments on each of the six questions featured on the questionnaire was included.

There are currently no publications on the use of providing video images of developing embryos to patients, and there are arguments for and against. A preliminary study considered patient feedback, and data were pooled from four CARE Fertility clinics. Since implementation of this online service in January 2013, 427 patients completed the questionnaire. This equated to 37 percent of those provided with a PIN for downloading the time-lapse images.

One question considered the timing of downloading the video images and asked whether patients viewed the video(s) straight after downloading, rather than saving for a specific point in their treatment journey (such as confirmation of pregnancy or following birth): 91 percent reported that they chose to view the images immediately, 3 percent disagreed, and free text comment suggested that a few patients would wait until their '12-week scan.' In terms of key motives for electing to use time lapse embryo selection, CAREmaps, patients were asked whether the opportunity to obtain video of their transferred embryo(s) was part of their decision making: 45 percent said that the video was not part of their decision making, and 31 percent said that it was. The free text comments from patients suggested that the uninterrupted culture of embryos and improved selection methods and clinical results were the key reasons for choosing this treatment option.

In order to assess the quality of information provided to patients, they were asked whether it was clear and aided their decision making: 85 percent stated that the information was clear, and 3 percent strongly disagreed and felt that they were still unclear as to what the treatment entailed and the proposed benefits of it.

Finally, patients were asked whether they would opt to use CAREmaps in a future treatment cycle. Of these patients, 93 percent stated that they would, 2 percent disagreed, and 5 percent had no opinion.

Despite the largely routine practice in IVF clinics worldwide of providing patients with photographic images of their preimplantation embryos, offering moving video images was considered to be a novel approach that required careful consideration, particularly as approximately half of those transferred embryos would not result in the birth of a baby. In order to minimize this risk of patient upset and in making assumptions about patient preferences, patient choice was provided within the download facility. By e-mailing a web link and unique patient PIN code to the patients, rather than showing them the video footage in the unit, patients could decide in their own time when and whether they wished to view their time-lapse video.

To date, there has been no negative feedback from over 2000 patients for whom we have utilized CAREmaps including patients who chose to view their videos. A selection of the free comments received is as follows:

> The video is amazing and really helps us to visually understand the development of the embryo in culture.

> We liked watching our embryos develop…it will be an amazing gift to our children if our treatment is successful.

> We have viewed the video and were very keen to do so. It was a fabulous opportunity to be able to see the embryos.

Two couples in particular have supported CARE Fertility in sharing their stories with other couples seeking assisted conception. Excerpts from their statements are presented below (see also Figures 19.1 and 19.2):

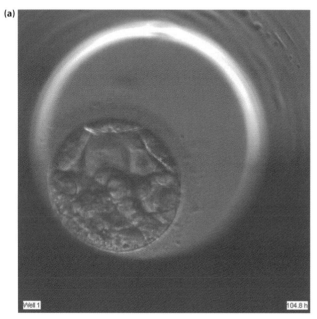

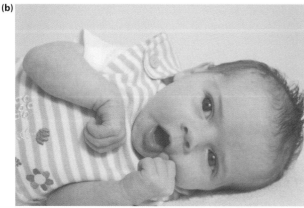

Figure 19.1 (a) Image of the embryo transferred which resulted in the birth of baby Isabella. (b) Baby Isabella. (Photograph reproduced with permission.)

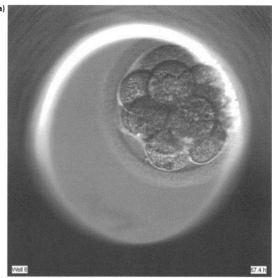

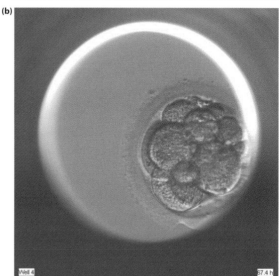

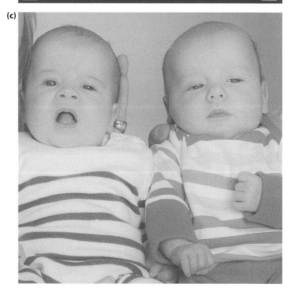

Figure 19.2 (a, b) The embryos transferred which resulted in the birth of babies Max and Barney. (c) Babies Max and Barney. (Photograph reproduced with permission.)

When the chance of having a family is ripped away from you, it is the worst thing imaginable. We were heartbroken and felt such a failure. We had got married, bought our first house, and now wanted a family…. The odds were stacked against us and we really feared it would never happen, but amazingly it worked first time and we are sure this new machine helped. She beat the odds and is our little miracle. We feel so privileged to be Isabella's mum and dad.

Gemma and Simon P, Wigan

Russ and I started trying for a family in 2010. Due to my 40th birthday fast approaching and having no luck trying to fall pregnant naturally, we turned to CARE for help. After numerous tests it was established there was nothing preventing us getting pregnant—but as time was against us we proceeded with a course of IVF.

We were lucky to have 13 eggs collected and two embryos were implanted after incubation and monitoring in the EmbryoScope. The result—a very enjoyable trouble-free twin pregnancy and we are thrilled to have our boys Max and Barney who were born on New Year's Eve.

We're delighted to have been involved in the development of the EmbryoScope; we can't wait to show the boys the video of them from the very beginning—such an amazing privilege very few ever get to see!

Anna H and Russell W, Cheshire

REFERENCE

1. Campbell A, Fishel S, Bowman N, et al. Modelling a risk classification of aneuploidy in human embryos using noninvasive morphokinetics. *Reprod Biomed Online*. 2013;26(5):477–485.

Index

A

Actomyosin cytoskeleton, 22, 25
Algorithms (*see also* models), 8–9, 115
Aneuploidy; *see also* Ploidy
    risk classification model, 8, 9
    risk variables, 16, 24, 43, 49
Annotations, 1
    consistency in, 9
    morphokinetic variables, 9
    subjectivity, 9–10
Assisted reproductive technology
        (ART), 39
Auxogyn (Eeva), 2, 3*f*

B

Binucleation, 75, 76*f*
Biomarkers, 8, 9
Blastocyst expansion, 59
Blastocyst hatching
    assistance methods, 59, 61
    biopsied *versus* nonbiopsied
            embryos, 61–62, 64
    expansion of fully hatched post
            biopsy, 63*f*
    multiple sites of, 61
    process, 59, 60–61*f*, 62–63*f*
    timing, 59
    transfer timing, 62
Blastocyst selection models, 16
Blastomeres
    direct cleavage from one to three, 8
    fusion, 69, 70*f*
    uneven, 8
Blastulation, 43, 49
    first signs of, 50*f*
    morphology variations, 55–57*f*
    prediction of, 8
    start time variations, 51–52*f*
    time to reach full blastulation,
            53–54*f*
Blighted ova, 41

C

Calcium oscillations, 22, 25
Calcium signaling, 71
CARE Fertility Group (UK), 14, 19, 115
CAREmaps, 115
Cell cycles, 13, 14*f*, 65
Cell divisions, synchronization, 13
Cell number, 7
Chorionicity, 8, 14

Chromosome abnormalities, 65, 75, 89;
        see also Aneuploidy
Cleavages
    direct, 7, 17, 65, 66*f*
    distribution of timings, 14
    identification with time-lapse
            technology, 7
    irregular, 7, 65, 68
    plane, 27
    rapid, 65, 67–68*f*
    reverse, 69, 70*f*
Clinical outcome measures, 8, 14
Compaction, 43, 44*f*
    fragmentation and, 34, 43
    incomplete, 43, 48*f*
    initiation, 44*f*, 45–47*f*, 45*f*
Computer servers, 10
Congenital abnormalities, 41
Consensus, 7, 9
Corona cells, 25, 61
Cryopreservation, 1, 7, 59, 65, 69
Culture
    dishes, 1, 2, 2*f*, 3
    environment, 1, 2, 7, 9, 14
    media, 9, 14
CultureCoins, 3, 5*f*
Cumulus cells, 25
Cytoplasm
    halos, 27
    inclusions, 79
    movements, 21, 22, 25

D

Data
    handling, 8
    median values, 8, 14, 16
    sharing, 10
    skewing, 14
    statistical analyses, 8, 10
Developmental milestones, 2, 8
Dextran serum supplement, 14
Diandric embryos, 41
Differentiation, first stage, 43
Digyny, 40*f*, 42
Diploid zygotes, 28, 39, 42
Direct cleavage, 7, 17, 65, 66*f*
DNA replication, 13, 28, 65

E

Eeva (Early Embryo Viability
        Assessment), 2, 3*f*
Embryo cell cycles, 13, 14*f*, 65

EmbryoScope, 3, 4*f*, 7, 10, 14
Embryo selection
    algorithms, 8–9
    exclusion criteria, 8, 39, 65, 79
    grading schemes, 7
    model transferability, 8–9
    morphological assessment and, 7, 8
    start point for model, 28
Embryo transfers
    multiple, data from, 8, 14
    timing of, 2, 62
Embryo viability, 2, 7; *see also*
        Embryo selection
    absence of zona, 61
    blastulation and, 8
    cell cycle durations, 13
    fragmentation and, 33, 43
Environmental stress, 7, 42
Esco (Miri), 3–4, 5*f*
Estradiol levels, 42, 71
Euploid embryos, 8
Exclusion criteria, 8
Expansion, of blastocyst, 59

F

Fertilization
    confirmation of, 25, 28, 39
    diandric, 41
    digynic, 39, 41, 42
    first visible manifestation of, 21
    normal *versus* abnormal, 21, 25, 39
    presence of sERC and, 71
    rate with granulation, 89
Fluorescent in situ hybridization
        (FISH), 39
Follicular response, excessive, 42
Folliculogenesis, susceptibility
        during, 69
Four-cell stage, multinucleation at, 8, 75
Fragmentation, 7, 33–34
    beginning at first cleavage
            division, 33*f*, 34
    exclusion at compaction stage, 36–37*f*
    inclusion at compaction stage, 35*f*
    localization, 34*f*
    in vivo, 33

G

Gas partial pressures, 9, 14
Gender, morphokinetics correlation, 19
Genetic fingerprinting, 8, 14
Genome activation events, 9

'Giant' oocytes, 42
Global IVF medium, 14
Golgi apparatus, 79
Granular cytoplasm, 89
    central, 89*f,* 90*f,* 91*f,* 92*f*
    embryo development with, 92*f,* 93*f*
    incidence, 93
    localized, 89*f,* 90*f,* 91*f*

H

Haploid zygotes, 39, 41
Hatching, *see* Blastocyst hatching

I

Immune protection, 59, 61
Implantation potential, 7
    blastomere fusion and, 69
    blastulation and, 49
    complete compaction and, 43
    late t2, 14
    presence of sERC, 69
    pronuclear fading, 28
    with rapid cleavage, 65
Imprinting disrorders, 71
Incubation
    dry, 3
    factors affecting outcome, 9
    uninterrupted, 7
Inner cell mass (ICM), 43, 49, 55–57*f*
Insemination timing, 28
Interphase, 13
Intracytoplasmic sperm
        injection (ICSI)
    blastocyst hatching and, 61
    damage to midpiece during, 65
    injection plane, 21
    outcome studies, 19, 22, 41, 89, 96
    time at insemination, 13
    unipronucleate fertilization, 39
    vacuolization and, 79
In vitro fertilization (IVF)
    clinics, 19, 115
    fragmentation and, 33
    hatching and, 59
    unipronucleate fertilization, 39
    zona defects and, 59, 96
Istanbul consensus workshop, 7

K

Known implantation data (KID),
    13–14, 15*f*

L

Live births, 116*f*
    aneuploidy and, 8, 9
    reverse cleavage and, 69
    triploidy in, 41

M

Maternal age, 9, 96
Mechanical stress, 7, 42
Metaphase II oocyte, 21*f*
Micronucleation, 75, 76*f*
Microscopy, static, 7
Microtubules, 25
Midpiece, 65
Miri, 3–4, 5*f*
Miscarriages, 41, 71
Mitosis
    cycle durations, 9
    phases, 13
    synchronicity, 9
Models, 8–9, 14
Monozygotic twinning, 14, 61
Morphokinetics
    criteria, 8
    gender and, 19
    terminology, 14
    variables, 9, 15*f*
Morphological assessment, 7, 9
Mosaics, 69
Multinucleation, 76*f,* 77*f*
    at four-cell stage, 8, 75
    and ploidy, 39, 41–42
    3PN, 21, 40*f,* 65
    5PN, 41*f*
    and reverse cleavage, 69

N

Novel events, 9

O

Oocyte microtubules, 25
Oocyte nuclear maturity, 21
Outcome measures, 8, 14

P

Parthogenesis, 39, 41
Partial hydatidiform moles, 41
Patient factors, 8, 9, 96
Patient feedback, 115–117
Perivitelline space, 25
Ploidy, 8, 16
    blastulation and, 49
    compaction and, 43
    of giant oocytes, 42
    number of pronuclei and, 39, 41–42
    PB2 alignment and, 24
Polar axis, 25, 27
Polar bodies (PB)
    adjacent and nonadjacent, 22, 23*f,* 24
    extrusion process, 21–22, 22*f,* 24
    failure of extrusion, 40*f,* 41–42
    morphology and outcomes, 24
    post extrusion movement, 23*f*

Polyploidy, 41, 42, 69
Polyspermy, 41, 59, 95
Pregnancy
    abnormalities, 39, 41
    loss, 14, 41, 71
    presence of sERC, 69, 71
    rates, 7, 24, 25, 62, 71, 89
    test as outcome data, 14
    vacuolation and, 79
    zona-free, 61
    ZP birefringence and, 95
Preimplantation genetic screening
    (PGS), 8
Primo Vision, 1–2, 2*f*
Pronuclei; *see also* Multinucleation
    appearance with extruded PBs, 22*f*
    asynchronous fading, 28, 30–31*f*
    dysmorphic, 28, 29*f*
    fading, 21, 28, 28*f*
    formation, 21, 22, 25, 26–27*f,* 27–28
    juxtaposition, 25, 27
    male *versus* female, 25
    morphology, 7, 25
    number of and ploidy, 39, 41–42
    premature fusion, 39, 41
    synchronous appearance, 27
    unipronucleate, 39, 41
Prophase, meiotic, 25

Q

Quality control, 9–10

R

Rapid cleavage, 65, 67–68*f*
Reannotation, 9
Receiver operating characteristic (ROC), 8
Reference images, 9
Refractile bodies, 79
Reverse cleavage, 69, 70*f*

S

Second cell cycle (cc2), 8, 17
Second opinions, 9
Smooth endoplasmic reticulum clusters
    (sERCs), 71–72, 73*f*
Smooth endoplasmic reticulum (SER), 79
Spermatozoa
    acrosome reaction, 95
    binding, 95
    centrosome, 25, 65
    nuclear envelope, 25
    penetration, 25, 41
    quality, 65
Sperm receptors, 95
S-phase, 13
Spindles
    formation, 65
    location, 22, 41

Standardized reporting, 7
Standard operating procedures (SOPs), 9, 10
Static microscopy, 1, 7, 8, 10, 65
Statistical analyses, 8, 10
Stimulation regimes, 71
Syngamy, 25, 28

T

Time-lapse imaging; *see also* Data
    applications of, 7, 10
    consensus, 7, 9
    current systems, 1–4, 5f
    flexibility, 10
    image storage, 9
    introduction of, 1, 7
    key elements of, 1
    opportunity and, 10
    patient viewing of video, 115–116
    standardized reporting, 7
    versus static assessment, 1, 7, 8, 10, 65
    systems comparison, 5t
    training in, 9
Time post insemination (t0), 13
Time to eight cells (t8), 16

Time to five cells (t5), 8, 16
Time to four cells (t4), 16
Time to full blastocyst stage (tB), 8, 16,
    17f, 49, 53–54f
Time to morula (tM), 13
Time to pronuclear fading (tPNf), 13
Time to start blastulation (tSB), 8, 16, 17f
Time to three cells (t3), 16
Time to two cells (t2), 14–15, 16f
Trinucleate zygotes, 21, 22f, 40f, 65
Triploid zygotes, 21, 22f, 40f, 41, 65
Trophectoderm (TE), 43, 49
    during blastocyst hatching, 59, 62f
    morphology variations, 55–57f

U

Unipronucleate (1PN) fertilization, 39, 41

V

Vacuolation, 79
    appearance at seven-cell stage, 85f
    change in number, 83f
    effect on oocyte competency, 87f

in later cleavage stages, 84f
in mature oocyte, 80f
in polar body, 86f
transient appearance, 81f
unchanged presence, 82f

Y

Y chromosomes, 39, 41

Z

Zoi server, 10
Zona breakers, 59
Zona hardening, 59
Zona pellucida binding protein (ZPBP), 95
Zona pellucida (ZP), 97–113f
    absence of, 61
    anomalies, 96
    birefringence, 95–96
    glycoproteins, 95
    hatching and, 59
    role of, 59, 95
    thickness, 95, 105f
Zygoticity, 8, 14